A Guide to Survivorship for Women
Who Have Ovarian Cancer

Dr. Robert E. Bristow is Director of Gynecologic Oncology Services, the Philip J. DiSaia Chair of Gynecologic Oncology, Chief of the Division of Gynecologic Oncology, and Professor of Obstetrics and Gynecology, University of California, Irvine.

Dr. Terri L. Cornelison is Associate Director for Clinical Research, Office of Research on Women's Health, Office of the Director, National Institutes of Health, and Assistant Professor of Gynecology and Obstetrics, Johns Hopkins Medical Institutions.

Dr. F. J. Montz was Professor of Gynecology and Obstetrics, Surgery, and Oncology, Johns Hopkins Hospital and Medical Institutions.

A Guide to Survivorship for Women Who Have Ovarian Cancer

second edition

Edited by

ROBERT E. BRISTOW, MD, MBA, FACOG, FACS

TERRI L. CORNELISON, MD, PhD, FACOG

F. J. MONTZ, MD, KM, FACOG, FACS

Johns Hopkins University Press

Baltimore

Note to the reader: This book is not meant to substitute for medical care of women with ovarian cancer, and treatment should not be based solely on its contents. Instead, treatment must be developed in a dialogue between the individual and her physician. Our book has been written to help with that dialogue.

Drug dosage: The author and publisher have made reasonable efforts to determine that the selection of drugs discussed in this text conform to the practices of the general medical community. The medications described do not necessarily have specific approval by the U.S. Food and Drug Administration for use in the diseases for which they are recommended. In view of ongoing research, changes in governmental regulation, and the constant flow of information relating to drug therapy and drug reactions, the reader is urged to check the package insert of each drug for any change in indications and dosage and for warnings and precautions. This is particularly important when the recommended agent is a new and/or infrequently used drug.

© 2005, 2015 Johns Hopkins University Press
All rights reserved. Published 2015
Printed in the United States of America on acid-free paper
9 8 7 6 5 4 3 2 1

The first edition of this book was published in 2005 as *A Guide to Survivorship for Women with Ovarian Cancer*, by F. J. Montz and Robert E. Bristow, with assistance from Paula J. Anastasia.

Johns Hopkins University Press
2715 North Charles Street
Baltimore, Maryland 21218-4363
www.press.jhu.edu

Library of Congress cataloging-in-publication data may be found on the final printed page of the book.

A catalog record for this book is available from the British Library.

Special discounts are available for bulk purchases of this book. For more information, please contact Special Sales at 410-516-6936 or specialsales@press.jhu.edu.

Johns Hopkins University Press uses environmentally friendly book materials, including recycled text paper that is composed of at least 30 percent post-consumer waste, whenever possible.

Contents

Tables

Foreword

More than fifteen years ago, three busy clinicians made a decision to write the first edition of this book as a way to help their patients survive ovarian cancer. Rick Montz, Rob Bristow, and Paula Anastasia made time in schedules that had no time because they believed that this book had to be written. They believed that there was information that every patient, family member, and friend needed to know about the journey of ovarian cancer.

Much has changed in those fifteen years. My husband, Rick Montz, died unexpectedly before his book was published, but he would have been honored by the praise it received. The time has come for the book to be updated, for new treatments to be discussed and new information to be presented. The purpose and heart of the book remain the same in this new edition, to bring information, support, and hope to women diagnosed with ovarian cancer. I know that Rick, Rob, and their colleague, Terri Cornelison, are grateful for the opportunity to help so many people and that they hope their readers are empowered by their work.

Kathleen Ryan, MD

A Guide to Survivorship for Women
Who Have Ovarian Cancer

Essential Concepts

F. J. Montz, MD, KM, FACOG, FACS

Survivorship

Numerous philosophers have spent numerous hours discussing the "life well lived." Most of them would agree that the well-lived life is full of love, experiences, sharing, meaningful relationships, accomplishments, and giving to others. As we all progress along this journey, our attempts to live the "well-lived life" are threatened by different forces, both internal (for example, disease) and external (for example, social pressures) to ourselves. Ovarian cancer is only one of many such threats to the life well lived. The sense of betrayal by one's own body, the strain on relationships, and the physical toll that the disease and its treatments may inflict are some of the challenges that ovarian cancer presents to living life well. Yet it is the deliberate and conscious choice to live life well that allows us to truly *survive* as we navigate the uncertainties of human life. That is what this book is about: *survivorship* in the face of, in spite of, and through ovarian cancer.

What do we mean by *survivorship?* Of course, part of survivorship is just that: outliving the disease and being around long enough to live out one's natural life expectancy and die of something else. Do you have to be totally free of ovarian cancer to be a survivor? Absolutely not. Does being totally free of any viable cancer cell constitute survivorship? An equally forceful "No." Many women die from their ovarian cancer within a relatively short span of years or months, but they survive the experience, being mentally, emotionally, and, within certain limits, physically intact. Similarly, we have had numerous patients who have survived the disease, strictly speaking, but whose lives have been in shambles in all other respects. One woman, the one who actually dies from her cancer, is a survivor; the other, the one who lives many years or even decades "disease-free," isn't. What makes the difference?

The difference is in being in control as much as possible; being as "well," in all aspects of wellness, as is possible; and finding joy and pleasure in ever having had a life well lived. Our mission, therefore, must be not to avoid death but to live life.

The Reality of Ovarian Cancer

Ovarian cancer can be viewed as three separate diseases. For some women, mainly those with early-stage disease and about 30 percent of women with advanced-stage disease, ovarian cancer is treated once and for all with an aggressive combination of surgery and chemotherapy. The disease is diagnosed, is treated, goes away, and never comes back.

Unfortunately, for a small but significant second group of women, the initial treatments fail, and the time from diagnosis to death is short—only months or little more than a year.

For most women, however, ovarian cancer is a chronic disease, one that is treated and goes into remission for a while and then returns, is retreated, goes back into remission, and so on. Eventually, perhaps years or decades from the time of initial diagnosis, the patient will succumb to the disease or to complications of its treatment. With this in mind, a greater emphasis is naturally placed on "what happens along the way," and the decisions made during these years or decades are enormously important.

Self-Determination

As we emphasize repeatedly in this book, we firmly believe that the patient must be informed, as much as possible and as much as she desires, about the disease and about the treatment options and their side effects and outcomes. We are unshakably committed to patient *self-determination*. For a woman to determine what she wants, however, she must know what the choices are and what the results of such choices are. It is our obligation, as health care providers, to meet our patients "where they are," to help them to prioritize their wishes and desires, and to develop *individualized* goals and agendas, while presenting them with the information they need to make decisions about what they do or don't want. Only after all these events have occurred can the well-informed patient have true self-determination.

Quality of Life

Another concept we repeatedly focus on in this book is that of *quality of life,* often abbreviated as QOL. Simply defined, quality of life is how well a person feels about everything she is and everything that makes up her universe. It includes measurable factors such as the amount of pain or physical discomfort she is experiencing, but it is much, much more than that. Emotional, psychological, sexual, spiritual factors—all of them difficult to measure—are part of QOL. For many of our patients, the nausea, loss of hair, and pain cause less suffering than do certain fears about the future: what is going to happen to the patient's three-year-old daughter, her frail life partner for whom she is the primary caregiver, or her own soul.

Issues of quality of life must be addressed daily, if not minute by minute, when making decisions regarding treatments and other interventions. Many women are willing to trade a marked deterioration in their measurable QOL for a significant chance of a cure or a meaningful prolonging of life; few are willing to do the same for only a few additional months or weeks. Unfortunately, patients often are not informed that they have choices or that QOL can play a role in decision making. We believe that quality-of-life issues are the most important issues our patients face in exercising self-determination. One of our primary goals in our medical practice and in this book is to empower women to wrestle with these issues.

CHAPTER 1

What Is Ovarian Cancer?

Terri L. Cornelison, MD, PhD, FACOG

O varian cancer is cancer that primarily involves or originates in the ovaries. Ovaries are pelvic structures, shaped like almonds, and are located on each side of the uterus. They are very important organs in the human female reproductive system. Normally functioning ovaries produce most of the human sex steroid hormones (*estrogen, progesterone,* and *androgens*); these substances control the start of puberty and sexual development and regulate the menstrual cycle. The ovaries are also the source of eggs (*oocytes*), which are released monthly (in the process of *ovulation*) in women of reproductive age. The ovaries of female babies already contain all the eggs they will ever have; as the girl matures, the hormones produced by her body cause the eggs to mature and to be released, ready for fertilization and growth into a fetus.

Most normal cells in the human body have a limited life span, which varies depending on their location in the body and the bodily functions they support. Normal cells are constantly being replaced. That is to say, in any normal tissue, some cells will be undergoing *cell suicide* (programmed cell death, or *apoptosis*), while new normal cells are being created to replace them. Cancer cells can turn off programmed cell death and thereby out-survive neighboring normal cells to form a *malignant tumor* (also called a *cancerous growth*). Cancer cells divide and reproduce more rapidly than normal cells and possess the capacity to spread to parts of the body located far away from the initial tumor (or *primary tumor*). When cancer cells spread in this fashion, the process is called *metastasis*. A *gynecologic malignancy* is a cancer that begins in the female reproductive organs. Ovarian cancer, in particular, represents the change of normal ovarian cells into a cancerous growth.

There are several different types of ovarian cancer. The most common type, *epithelial ovarian cancer,* also called ovarian *carcinoma,* looks like cells derived from the lining, or surface (*epithelium*), of the ovary. A carcinoma is a cancer derived from an epithelium. Epithelial ovarian cancer is generally described in terms of two parameters. The first parameter is called the *histology* (cell subtype) and is based on what the cells look like under the microscope (for example, *serous, mucinous, endometrioid,* or *clear* cells). The second parameter is called the *degree of differentiation* (or *grade*): are the cells well differentiated, moderately differentiated, or poorly differentiated? The degree of differentiation refers to how closely the cancer cells resemble normal, noncancerous cells. Well-differentiated (*low-grade*) cancer cells look very much like normal cells, while poorly differentiated (*high-grade*) cells do not resemble normal cells at all.

What researchers are coming to understand is that epithelial ovarian cancer is not just one disease but actually many different types of cancers, based on histology and grade. These various types of ovarian cancer can be categorized into two groups, one group designated Type I, the other Type II.[1] Type I tumors include low-grade serous, low-grade endometrioid, clear cell, and mucinous cancers. Type II tumors include high-grade serous, high-grade endometrioid, and undifferentiated (no discernable histologic subtype). Type II tumors represent 75 percent of all epithelial ovarian carcinomas, and high-grade serous is the most common.[2]

Other, less common, types of ovarian cancer include *germ cell tumors* and *sex-cord stromal tumors,* which begin deep inside the ovary. These types of ovarian cancer are also known as *non-epithelial ovarian cancers.* Germ cell tumors arise from the egg-producing cells in the ovary; sex-cord stromal tumors come from the cells surrounding the egg-producing cells (the fibrous connective tissue, or supporting stroma).

For most women, the overall lifetime risk of developing ovarian cancer is small: less than 1 in 71.[3] And ovarian cancer is not the most common gynecologic malignancy—endometrial cancer is. The sad truth, however, is that ovarian cancer is the most lethal gynecologic malignancy. In the United States, even though ovarian cancer represents only 28 percent of new gynecologic cancer cases, it accounts for more deaths than all other gynecologic malignancies combined and remains the fifth leading cause of all cancer-related deaths.[4] Each year, approximately 22,000 women are diagnosed with ovarian cancer in this country, and more than 14,300 women die from this disease.[3] Ninety percent of ovarian cancer deaths are caused by Type II tumors.[2]

Although these numbers are saddening, it is important to put them into perspective. The most common cause of death for American women isn't cancer at all; it is heart and blood vessel (*cardiac* and *peripheral vascular*) diseases. Almost one-third of all American women die from heart and blood vessel disease (30.7%).[5] That translates to 395,808 women a year! It has been proved and is widely accepted by the medical community that the most common causes of cardiovascular diseases are related to a person's lifestyle. Obesity, inactivity, high-fat diets, smoking—all increase the risk of developing these diseases.

The most common cause of cancer-related death for American women is also directly linked to lifestyle: lung cancer. Annually, more than 108,000 women in the United States are diagnosed with this disease, and over 72,300 women die from lung cancer, most of them as a result of a cancer induced by cigarette smoking. Breast cancer is the most common cancer in American women, affecting more than 232,600 women each year. Fortunately, most women with breast cancer (85 to 90 percent) survive this disease. Much of the success in breast cancer treatment is the result of early diagnosis, thanks to the wide implementation of mammograms. The other major cause of cancer mortality in American women is colon cancer, a malignancy that is also strongly related to lifestyle. Cigarette smoking, a diet low in fruits and vegetables, and reduced levels of physical activity are associated with an increased risk of colon cancer. Colon cancer, too, can be diagnosed early, with stool *occult* (invisible) blood testing and *colonoscopy* (looking at the inside of the large intestine with a lighted telescope).

Origin of Ovarian Cancer

Despite decades of research, the origin of epithelial ovarian cancer is still poorly understood. Where does this cancer come from? It was always assumed, and quite reasonably so, that ovarian cancer originates in the ovary. This was because when the cancer was detected, most often at an advanced stage, the ovary was entirely involved. Yet numerous investigators have carefully examined the ovaries for precancer (*precursor*) lesions, and no verifiable lesions have ever been found.[1]

The traditional view was that ovarian cancer is a result of incessant ovulation, which occurs when a woman releases at least one egg from her ovaries each month for a great many months.[1] Some ovarian epithelial cells were believed to undergo *metaplasia* (change in form) into cells that resembled the epithelia of the fallopian tube, lining of the uterus (*endometrium*), lining of the cervical canal (*endocervix*), gastrointestinal tract, and urinary bladder. Ovulation then led to trapping of these metaplastic cells in the ovary, forming inclusion cysts; "incessant ovulation" accompanied by an ongoing repetitive wound-healing process led to epithelial ovarian cancer.

It is true that early *menarche* (starting of menstruation), late *menopause* (stopping of menstruation), few or no pregnancies, no breast-feeding—all increase the total number of ovulations in a woman's lifetime. Each time the ovary releases an egg (*ovulation*), the surface of the ovary ruptures (to release the egg). This process of rupture results in trauma to the surface of the ovary, which is then repaired by new ovarian surface cells. It was thought that this repeated trauma and repair might result in an increased risk of ovarian cancer since *genetic mutations* (abnormalities) might occur during the repair process. This incessant ovulation theory was conventionally accepted because surface epithelial inclusion cysts are often found in the ovary. But again, no verifiable precursor lesions have been found in these cysts, and women with inclusion cysts do not have an increased risk for ovarian cancer.[6]

Recent discoveries in women with inherited high risk for ovarian cancer seem to indicate that high-grade serous ovarian cancers may originate in the fallopian tube and then spread to the ovarian surface. The BRCA1 and BRCA2 genes have been linked to the development of ovarian cancer. When women with BRCA1/2 mutations underwent surgical removal of their fallopian tubes and ovaries to prevent ovarian cancer (*prophylactic salpingo-oophorectomy*), precursor lesions and small early serous cancers were detected in the fallopian tubes.[7-14] These tubal cancers were histologically identical to serous ovarian cancer. In addition, the precursor lesions, found in approximately 80 percent of fallopian tube specimens from women with BRCA1/2 mutations,[15] are also associated with 70 percent of nonhereditary (*sporadic*) advanced serous ovarian cancer.[16] Further investigations are being done to determine if the fallopian tube is truly the site of origin for high-grade serous ovarian cancer.

Endometrioid and clear cell ovarian cancers are hypothesized to arise from endometrial tissue implanted on the ovary (*endometriosis*). This is supported by well-documented identification of transitional areas of endometriosis that contain the full range from *benign* (noncancer) to atypical cells located next to areas of ovarian cancer. Also, epidemiological studies show that the risk of ovarian cancer among women with endometriosis is higher, by 30 to 40 percent, than among women without endometriosis.[17]

Thus, it would appear that high-grade serous ovarian cancers may originate in the fallopian tubes, while low-grade serous ovarian cancers may arise from the ovarian surface epithelium.[1] Endometrioid and clear cell ovarian cancers may arise from endometrial tissue implants.[1] The cell origin of mucinous ovarian cancer remains unclear.

Risk Factors

We know some factors that place a woman at higher-than-average risk of developing ovarian cancer. Table 1.1 lists these risk factors. Early menarche, late menopause, few or no pregnancies, no

TABLE 1.1   *Risk Factors for Ovarian Cancer*

Risk Factor	Increased Relative Risk*
Family history of ovarian cancer†	3 to 4 times
Older age	3 times
North American or European descent	2 to 5 times
Infertility	2 to 5 times
Nulligravid (no pregnancies)	2 to 3 times
High socioeconomic status	1.5 to 2 times
Late menopause	1.5 to 2 times
Early menarche	1.5 times

SOURCE: Brinton LA, Lacey Jr JV, Sherman ME, "Epidemiology of Gynecologic Cancers," in Hoskins WJ, Perez CA, Young RC, Barakat RR, Markman M, Randall ME, *Principles and Practice of Gynecologic Oncology*, 4th ed. (Baltimore: Lippincott Williams and Wilkins, 2005): 3–32.

*Relative to the risk for women without the risk factor.

†In a first-degree relative (for example, a mother) or a second-degree relative (for example, an aunt).

breastfeeding, not using birth control pills (oral contraceptive pills, or OCPs)—all are associated with an increased risk for ovarian cancer. Though all these factors increase the total number of ovulations in a woman's lifetime, incessant ovulation may not necessarily be the underlying mechanism for the increased risk. Investigators are currently evaluating the role of incessant ovulation and the effect this may have on the fallopian tube in view of evidence that high-grade serous ovarian cancers may originate in the fallopian tube.

Another factor that plays an important role in developing ovarian cancer is the balance between local (ovarian) concentrations of the sex steroid hormones estrogen and progesterone, called the *hormonal milieu*. A shift in this balance from the normal progesterone-dominant hormonal milieu to one of relative progesterone deficiency has been associated with an increased risk of ovarian cancer. As we* discuss below, progesterone, which inhibits ovulation, seems to be effective at decreasing (though not eliminating) the risk of ovarian cancer in more ways than one.

The most significant risk factor, however, is a family history of ovarian cancer and the associated genetic predisposition for devel-

* Although some of the chapters in this book are written by individual authors, the voice ("we") used throughout is that of all medical professionals who contributed to this volume.

oping the disease. A family history of ovarian cancer in a first-degree relative (a mother or a sister) or a second-degree relative (an aunt or a grandmother) makes a woman three or four times more likely to develop ovarian cancer. Several potential genetic abnormalities can lead to an increased risk for and eventual development of ovarian cancer. Most human cancers develop as a result of abnormalities (or mutations) in certain genes.

Genes are the functional units of heredity; each gene is located at a specific site on a chromosome. *Oncogenes* are genes that, when activated (by a mutation, for example), cause uncontrolled cell growth and produce a malignant tumor. Another group of genes, called *tumor suppressor genes,* normally function to prevent cancerous growths. When a tumor suppressor gene suffers a mutation, this normal preventive function is lost, and a cancer develops. For example, the BRCA1 and BRCA2 genes, located on chromosomes 17 and 13, respectively, are both tumor suppressor genes. Mutations in these genes that block normal gene function lead to the development of ovarian cancer as well as breast cancer. At most, however, only 10 to 15 percent of all ovarian cancers are the result of a known genetic predisposition. Genetic predisposition may be associated with a similar increased risk of developing breast cancer. The genetic abnormalities are more common in women of Eastern European Jewish descent (so-called Ashkenazi Jews). If the *lifetime risk* of ovarian cancer is defined as the possibility that a woman will develop ovarian cancer before living out her natural life of eighty-plus years, then in some women with these genes, the lifetime risk may be as high as 35 to 46 percent.[18] Women such as these may benefit greatly from participating in some form of screening (screening is discussed later in this chapter).

In addition to family history and genetic predisposition, increasing age, infertility (despite ovulation), and certain demographic characteristics (high socioeconomic status) are associated with an increased risk of ovarian cancer.

Prevention

We have identified factors that put a woman at increased risk for developing ovarian cancer. Now we can discuss how a woman might decrease the risk. Obviously, we can't change who her parents were or when she naturally starts and stops menstruating. But there are ways to decrease risk. It is unreasonable to encourage women to become pregnant or to breastfeed just to decrease their risk of ovarian cancer because, as noted, the overall risk for the average woman is small. But it may be reasonable for women at increased risk for ovarian cancer to use OCPs as their means of birth control, particularly if they have a family history of ovarian cancer. Using birth control pills may be a reasonable approach for risk reduction in some women; however, no clinical trial has been done to prove this.

There is growing evidence that taking exogenous progesterone (that is, progesterone not produced by the body), particularly in relatively high doses for a short time or lower doses for a longer time, protects against ovarian cancer better than the approach of preventing ovulation alone. Progesterone appears to be effective at stimulating "suicide" by cells that have undergone the genetic and molecular changes that could lead to developing ovarian cancer. This is an exciting finding, as it may offer an easy and low-risk way to decrease a woman's chance of developing ovarian cancer. Women at high risk for ovarian cancer, however, tend to also be at high risk for breast cancer. In particular, women who are BRCA1/2 mutation carriers have a 47 to 66 percent lifetime risk for developing breast cancer.[18] Findings from the Women's Health Initiative study indicate that progesterone increases the risk for breast cancer.[19] We will want to see the results of thorough scientific testing with a progesterone formulation that does not increase breast cancer risk before encouraging women to take progesterone as a means of preventing ovarian cancer.

What about removing the ovaries as a way to protect against this frequently lethal disease? A procedure called *prophylactic oophorectomy* can be done, in which a woman's ovaries are removed even though the ovaries are apparently healthy. This procedure may be offered to women with inherited high risk for ovarian cancer.

In most cases, prophylactic oophorectomy can be performed using minimally invasive surgical techniques. Minimally invasive surgery, also known as *laparoscopy*, involves the use of a small fiberoptic scope (the *laparoscope*) and small surgical instruments introduced into the abdominal cavity through three or four incisions that are 5 to 10 millimeters in size. The laparoscopic approach to prophylactic oophorectomy is associated with less pain and a shorter postoperative recovery time than the traditional approach via *laparotomy* (a larger incision in the abdomen). Some laparoscopic surgeries may be done with robotic assistance. Nevertheless, even minimally invasive surgery is not entirely without risk. The chance of dying during surgery is 1 in 1,500, and 1 to 2 women out of 100 will have a major, life-threatening complication. The risk of having a major complication is about the same as the risk for the average woman of ever developing ovarian cancer. Therefore, it does not make sense for women of average risk to remove the ovaries to prevent ovarian cancer.

The ovaries provide 95 percent of a woman's estrogen, so even for women who have a higher than 1 or 2 percent chance of developing ovarian cancer, there are significant concerns about what happens when the ovaries are removed. Estrogen is a hormone that a woman's body relies on to keep nearly every organ working at its best. The potential problems with prophylactic oophorectomies are much greater for premenopausal women than for postmenopausal women. Beyond the simple but important quality-of-life side effects of an early (before the age of 45) surgical menopause, the average woman's life is shortened by removing her ovaries early if she doesn't take adequate doses of estrogen replacement.

Why shouldn't postmenopausal women who are at increased risk have prophylactic oophorectomies? The problem is that women who are at increased risk because of a genetic predisposition have about a 25 percent chance of developing ovarian cancer before they reach their mid-forties, so the real benefit for having a prophylactic oophorectomy is when the woman is premenopausal. In addition, many of these same women are also at increased risk of developing breast cancer. Women who have a higher-than-average risk of developing breast cancer, and women who have had breast cancer, may choose not to take hormone replacement therapy—therapy that is often desirable after removal of the ovaries. A woman who is facing these complex and difficult issues needs to consult a gynecologic oncologist who is well versed in the scientific data, a skilled and open communicator, and an expert in performing laparoscopic surgery. Studies are being planned to evaluate if prophylactic salpingectomy (removal of the fallopian tubes) alone can prevent high-grade serous ovarian cancer; however, this procedure will not protect these women from breast cancer.

We strongly encourage any woman who is at increased risk of developing ovarian cancer because of personal variables (as described above), or because she has even one relative with verified ovarian cancer, to seek out the expertise of a gynecologic oncologist and discuss these complex issues.

Screening

In the United States, people who see a doctor for a regular checkup will be routinely screened for any number of diseases—breast cancer with mammography, cervical cancer with the Pap test and the human papillomavirus (HPV) test, and prostate cancer with blood prostate-specific antigen (PSA) determination, just to name a few. But routine screening is only possible if it is cost effective, and a cost-effective screening program for any specific disease is only possible under the following conditions: (1) the disease must be a common source of *morbidity* (illness) and mortality in the group to be screened; (2) there must be a precursor, preinvasive, or early invasive disease state that can be treated to prevent the development of either a crippling or a lethal malignancy; and (3) there must be a method of screening that is easy and that poses little risk for the patient.

Ovarian cancer doesn't fulfill all these requirements. The disease is not a *common* source of illness and death for women in the United States—not common enough to justify the expense of a broad-based screening program, in any case. For years the existence of a preinvasive, or early, ovarian cancer remained unproven, and therefore no such "early disease" could be identified by a screening or early-detection tool. Similarly, there are no reliable screening tools available for women at average risk that are *sensitive* enough to detect almost all ovarian cancers and *specific* enough to detect only ovarian cancer (and not benign conditions). Fortunately, advances in screening for ovarian cancer have been made, and studies have shown that new methods, or newer ways to use old methods, can identify some ovarian cancers early. Currently, ovarian cancer is detected through physical assessment and presence of symptoms, a blood test for the tumor marker CA-125, and imaging methods such as transvaginal ultrasound.

CA-125 (cancer antigen 125, or carbohydrate antigen 125) was first described in 1981, and it remains the most widely studied tumor marker for ovarian cancer. It is a *glycoprotein* (sugar and protein molecule) normally expressed (present) on the surface of the ovary, but it is also expressed on the lining of the fallopian tubes, uterus, and cervix, as well as on the surface of the entire abdominal cavity, all organs within the abdominal cavity, the lung cavity, and the heart cavity. Since CA-125 is highly glycosylated, it attracts water molecules and creates a lubricating barrier on the cell surface against foreign particles and infectious agents.

CA-125 is elevated in 78 percent of advanced epithelial ovarian cancers. The challenge with CA-125 is that it is also elevated in a number of other conditions, such as pregnancy, fibroids, endometriosis, cirrhosis, pancreatitis, and pneumonia. CA-125 is located on so many surfaces in the body that any irritation (e.g., by foreign particles, infectious agents, tissue injury, tissue growth) on these other surfaces will cause an elevated CA-125 level, which is produced to protect the cell against the irritant. So an elevated CA-125 is not very specific to ovarian cancer, and 20 percent of elevated CA-125 levels are in women who do not have cancer. Another challenge with CA-125 is that it is elevated in only half of early ovarian cancers and therefore is not a good test to detect early disease, particularly in women with average risk for disease.

In women with an inherited high risk for ovarian cancer, however, a steady rise in the CA-125 level over time is a better predictor for ovarian cancer than just an isolated CA-125 level. One approach to improve CA-125 performance as a marker is to develop a more sophisticated use of CA-125. An example of this is the Risk of Ovarian Cancer Algorithm (ROCA), which is based on a series of CA-125 measurements drawn at regular intervals. When the ROCA score exceeds a 1 percent risk of having ovarian cancer, patients are to undergo transvaginal ultrasound to determine whether additional intervention is warranted. This strategy is currently being studied by the Gynecologic Oncology Group (now a part of NRG Oncology) as well as in a parallel trial being conducted by the National Cancer Institute's Cancer Genetics Network, and results are expected in the next few years. In the meantime, women with inherited high risk for ovarian cancer may be followed (screened) with CA-125 levels looking for an absolute elevated value or a rise in even a normal value over time.

Transvaginal ultrasound is an imaging method that has been used to screen for ovarian cancer in women at high risk for disease. The ultrasound uses sound waves to evaluate the ovaries for any changes in volume (size) and *morphology* (shape) that may indicate an early ovarian cancer. Transvaginal imaging allows for the closest and most accurate depiction of the ovaries. It can be used to pick up subtle cancerous changes in the ovaries and potentially allow for diagnosis and surgical removal before the disease has had a chance to spread. This method is easy to perform, well accepted, and relatively cost effective. The challenge is inconsistent reliability for the ultrasound to distinguish benign cysts from cancerous growths. Newer technologies such as three-dimensional (3D) ultrasonography may be worth investigating. Before considering surgical removal of the ovaries because of an abnormal finding on an ultrasound, a woman should make sure that the ultrasound study has been reviewed by a radiologist with expertise in ovarian imaging and should consult with a gynecologic oncologist to discuss the results, the risks and benefits of surgery, and other options that may be appropriate (continued observation, for example).

Another approach to improve performance of the CA-125 and ultrasound is to combine them in a bimodal screening strategy.[20] For example, if the CA-125 is elevated, then a transvaginal ultrasound is obtained. Screening trials have shown that transvaginal ultrasound can reduce the rate of false positive tests by tenfold among women with a positive CA-125 test. This bimodal strategy is being evaluated in the United Kingdom and here in the United States.

Magnetic resonance imaging (MRI) and *positron emission tomography* (PET) are other imaging tests used to diagnose ovarian cancer. Just like CA-125 and transvaginal ultrasound, however, these tests are not sensitive enough or specific enough to be used for ovarian cancer screening in the general population.[21,22]

Even with improvements in these screening methods, there is

still the problem of determining which women are at *enough* of an increased risk to justify the expense of repeated ultrasounds, evaluation, and subsequent management of changes that have produced no symptoms and are most likely nonmalignant. For example, a woman with no family history of ovarian cancer and limited personal risk factors is unlikely to develop ovarian cancer in her lifetime. It is difficult to endorse routine screening in this case, because the expense and potential for personal anxiety associated with screening outweigh the small likelihood of detecting an early ovarian cancer. As with the issue of prophylactic oophorectomy, this issue requires the assessment of a woman's personal risk of developing ovarian cancer and her concerns regarding that risk. This sort of assessment is best completed by health care professionals skilled at risk determination and counseling.

We are fortunate to have such a group of individuals at the Johns Hopkins Hospital and Medical Institutions. These professionals work in concert with us in what is called the BOSS (Breast and Ovarian Surveillance Service), and we are all part of the Ovarian Cancer Network, a group of individuals who perform clinical trials investigating screening for and prevention of ovarian cancer. We routinely refer to BOSS any of our patients who have questions regarding their individual risk of ovarian or breast cancer. If nothing else (and most frequently this is the case), patients are comforted when they find out that their risk for ovarian cancer is much lower than they had anticipated and that there is no need for intervention.

At this time, no screening methods perform well enough to be used in women with average risk for ovarian cancer. For women with an inherited high risk for this disease, a screening strategy that uses a combination of CA-125 and transvaginal ultrasound is a reasonable approach.

Symptoms and Diagnosis

One reason ovarian cancer can be a difficult disease to cure is that it has often spread extensively by the time it is diagnosed. Another reason is that the treatments do not work completely for everyone. But the fact that the disease so often spreads before it is diagnosed helps to illustrate the point that there are no *unique* symptoms and few *unique* findings upon examination or laboratory testing for ovarian cancer that can lead a health care professional to make a definite diagnosis very early. The idea that ovarian cancer is a "silent killer" has been proved a myth, however. The vast majority of women with either early or late disease do have some presenting symptoms. (The term *presenting symptoms* is doctor-speak for whatever caused a person to seek medical attention in the first place—for example, a cough, fatigue, or pain.)

Women with epithelial ovarian cancer may present with bloating, abdominal or pelvic pain, urinary urgency or frequency, difficulty eating or feeling full, which are the same symptoms that occur in many gastrointestinal disorders.[23] Epithelial ovarian cancer should be suspected, however, when these symptoms coexist with other symptoms, occur almost daily, and are more severe than expected. Unfortunately, all too frequently, these symptoms are either ignored by the patient or inadequately evaluated by the woman's health care provider.

Almost one-third of women who are eventually diagnosed with ovarian cancer experienced their symptoms for more than six months before the diagnosis was made. *This is unacceptable.* We encourage women to visit their health care provider when new symptoms persist. And if a woman's health care provider doesn't evaluate the symptom to the woman's satisfaction, she needs to demand further evaluation or even get a new health care provider. You have no better health advocate than yourself, and you need to make sure that your concerns are addressed adequately.

The common presenting symptoms of ovarian cancer, as reported by women with this disease, are listed in table 1.2. To a lesser or greater degree, they are present in all of us. Furthermore, these symptoms are associated with numerous other medical problems that are common in women in the age group in which ovarian cancer most frequently occurs—women in their sixties and seventies. Other such medical problems include stool habit changes (often as a result of medications or dietary changes) and *diverticulitis* (inflammation of the large intestine as a result of small hernias in its muscle wall).

These symptoms are quite common and are often just part of

TABLE 1.2   *Symptoms of Ovarian Cancer*

Symptom	Frequency (percent)
Increased abdominal size	61
Abdominal bloating	57
Fatigue	47
Abdominal pain	36
Indigestion	31
Frequent urination	27
Pelvic pain	26
Constipation	25
Incontinence of urine	24
Back pain	23
Pain with intercourse	17
Inability to eat normally	16
Palpable mass	14
Vaginal bleeding	13

SOURCE: Goff BA, Mandel L, Muntz HG, Melancon CH, "Ovarian carcinoma diagnosis," *Cancer* 89 (2000): 2068–2075.

being middle aged or older. That is why many women who develop these symptoms put off visiting a health care professional. And when a woman with these symptoms does see her health care provider, it is difficult for the medical professional to determine how aggressive to be in attempting to find out exactly what is going on. Not uncommonly, there is no rush to find the source of the symptoms—and an additional delay occurs, this time brought about by the health care provider. The prudent medical professional will make sure that a patient is up to date in her screening tests for cancer of the cervix (Pap smear, HPV), breast (mammography), and colon (colonoscopy). For most women, this screening will include, in addition to a mammogram, a recent sigmoidoscopy or colonoscopy (looking inside the large intestine to see if there are any abnormal growths). A thorough pelvic examination is a critical but unfortunately often excluded part of these evaluations.

A symptom index is being developed to aid clinicians in evaluating women for early symptoms of epithelial ovarian cancer. The symptom index is considered to be positive if a woman reports any of the following symptoms that are (1) new to her within the past year and (2) occur more than twelve times per month: pelvic or abdominal pain, increased abdominal size or abdominal bloating, difficulty eating or feeling full quickly.[24] In one study, when women were screened with the symptom index and followed up with CA-125 and transvaginal ultrasound for a positive index, no major (laparoscopy or laparotomy) unindicated procedures resulted.[25] Further validation studies are needed for this index, and it is not yet recommended for routine clinical use.

Based on the degree of symptoms that a woman may have and her underlying risk of developing ovarian cancer, further investigations such as transvaginal ultrasounds and other imaging studies (CT scan [computed tomography] or MRI) may be warranted. However, little time should be spent performing multiple additional studies that are remarkably inaccurate and potentially expensive and that can lead to delays in diagnosis and treatment. If a mass is detected and CA-125 is elevated, or if a mass is persistent even if CA-125 is normal, then surgical evaluation is warranted. This surgery may involve only removal of the mass if there is a low suspicion of malignancy, or removal of the mass, ovary, and fallopian tube. If ovarian cancer is discovered, a gynecologic oncologist should be available to consult during the surgery, so that the appropriate surgical procedure to determine the extent (*stage*) of the cancer and to fully remove the cancer can be done at once to maximize the woman's potential for survival. It has been shown that survival from ovarian cancer is improved when optimal removal of the disease is performed at the time of the initial surgery.

In this chapter we have described the current state of knowledge about the origin of ovarian cancer, risk factors for ovarian cancer, and possible preventive measures and diagnostic tests for the disease. It is always preferable, but not always possible, to prevent disease. When a woman develops ovarian cancer, optimal treatment is based on the triad of (1) appropriate and aggressive surgery, (2) state-of-the-art chemotherapy, and (3) comprehensive care for the needs of the patient and the people who are important to her. In the chapters that follow, we discuss in detail these three approaches to treatment.

A Personal Perspective on Surgery

Annette Mattern

I've had numerous surgeries in my twenty-eight years of survivorship. Most were to remove tumors; some were secondary, as a result of treatments or prior surgeries. My initial surgery, as with many ovarian cancer cases, was the result of a visit to the ER, so it was completely out of my hands. Fortunately, a gynecologic oncologist was called in immediately to deal with a ruptured ovarian mass. However, many subsequent trips to the operating room have given me some insights on preparing for and recovering from surgery.

Plan ahead. I plan for surgeries because I know they are inevitable and, for ovarian cancer, are usually very invasive. Surgery will always involve anesthesia, so prior to surgery, I practice daily yogic breathing to prepare my lungs. I also focus on a strict anti-inflammatory diet to reduce any impediments to healing. A great resource is an oncology-certified nutritionist who can help you customize a nutrition plan that reduces inflammation while supporting your personal situation. I try to arrange for home support that will be needed during recovery, such as for restocking stool softeners and other over-the-counter drugs. I prepare my living space, mindful of safety issues that could be a serious problem, such as loose rugs and overzealous pets.

Prepare your team. Friends and family will offer to help but will wait for direction from you. I've found that creating a rough calendar and assigning duties makes it easier on everyone. Neighbors get a house key to allow easier access while others may be responsible for bringing groceries or providing transportation. I've found it's better to overplan and scale back than to scramble at the last minute when you need help. And always have contact numbers handy for you and accessible to caregivers.

Educate yourself. Know the signs of infection and what symptoms might be cause for concern. Understand the side effects of your medications. Abdominal surgery is painful, but pain meds cause constipation, so plan with your nurse how and when to transition off pain medication—or any medication—and report any concerns you may have before the problem becomes worse.

Keep your perspective. Know that you are on a path to recovery. I commit myself to everything that will keep my mind calm and support the miracle of healing that my body is going through. I surround myself with positive and uplifting people, messages, and energy. I remind myself of all that I am grateful for and repeat it over and over again.

Choose the right surgeon. All board-certified gynecologic oncologists are surgeons, so they should always be the leader of the surgical team working on your case, even if other specialists are called in to help. Statistics prove that ovarian cancer patients who are operated on by gynecologic oncologists have a better survival rate. When selecting my surgeon, I sought a doctor with experience in my particular subtype of ovarian cancer, and I believe that is why I am a survivor today.

CHAPTER 2

Surgery for Ovarian Cancer

Robert E. Bristow, MD, MBA, FACOG, FACS, and
F. J. Montz, MD, KM, FACOG, FACS

A t first glance, surgery may seem to be a straightforward concept: a problem exists, and the person has an operation to fix
it. In fact, however, surgery is a complex process beginning well before the actual operation and extending for some time after recovery.
Surgery for ovarian cancer is no exception. The extent of surgery will
necessarily vary by the particular type of ovarian cancer, the extent
of disease, and the patient's overall medical condition as well as her
individual goals for treatment.

The specific tests ordered to diagnose ovarian cancer, the procedures performed to treat it, and even the manner in which the surgery is carried out may be different in different medical institutions
and even among different surgeons, depending on the physician's
experience and judgment. This chapter presents one view of the most
important issues surrounding surgery for ovarian cancer as it stands
today. Other health care providers may recommend approaches that
are different from the perspective presented here—and we want the
reader to recognize this fact, too. Different approaches may be just
as appropriate as the approach represented in this chapter. Furthermore, as technology continues to advance and more research is con-

ducted, certain aspects of the treatment program described in this book will be refined, and some of the approaches described here may even become outdated.

Diagnostic Tests

When a woman visits a health care provider because she is experiencing symptoms, the health care provider will probably recommend a series of diagnostic tests to determine the cause of the symptoms. Ovarian cancer, as noted in chapter 1, shares symptoms with other health problems, such as diverticulitis. When a patient describes symptoms that could signal a number of different problems, the health care provider will create a mental list of possible diagnoses. This process is called making a *differential diagnosis*. Tests are performed to rule out or confirm the diagnoses on the list. As test results become known, one of the potential diagnoses becomes most likely, and then further testing can focus intently on ruling out or confirming that specific diagnosis.

Many women who are ultimately diagnosed with ovarian cancer initially visit their health care provider and describe somewhat vague, or nonspecific, symptoms, and then are found to have an ovarian cyst or mass (also referred to as an *adnexal mass*), usually detected on a pelvic ultrasound or CT (computed tomography) scan. These imaging tests can reveal that there is an abnormality in the ovary or ovaries, but the tests are not always able to indicate whether that abnormality represents a cancer. Certain features of an adnexal mass increase the level of suspicion for ovarian cancer: solid areas, thick septations (a piece of tissue dividing one big cyst into two smaller cysts), internal vegetations (or growths), and ascites (or fluid in the abdomen). But even these features are not 100 percent accurate in predicting the diagnosis.

To get a more accurate indication of the diagnosis, clinicians will often rely on blood tests, known as serum biomarkers, to (1) better characterize the likelihood of ovarian cancer (either low or high risk) and (2) help decide whether the patient should be referred to a gynecologic oncologist for surgery (if she is at high risk for ovarian cancer) or whether she can just as well have surgery performed by a general gynecologist or noncancer specialist (if she is at low risk for ovarian cancer). These are critical distinctions, because gynecologic oncologists are specifically trained in the surgical management of ovarian cancer, and multiple scientific research studies have shown that these specialists are more likely to perform a proper staging operation or complete debulking surgery than other types of surgeons.

The serum CA-125 level has been used most often as a biomarker for ovarian cancer risk. Although CA-125 can be a useful marker for diagnosing advanced-stage ovarian cancer, it is neither sensitive enough (able to detect true cancer cases) nor specific enough (able to exclude noncancer cases) for predicting the diagnosis for women with early-stage ovarian cancer when used as an isolated test. Because of these uncertainties, the American College of Obstetricians and Gynecologists (ACOG) and the Society of Gynecologic Oncology (SGO) have jointly published guidelines for when referral to a gynecologic oncologist is indicated; these guidelines can help physicians decide which specialty of physician is most appropriate to perform surgery for an ovarian mass. The Risk of Malignancy Index (RMI) is a decision support algorithm for clinicians, which has been updated several times since it was originally proposed in the 1990s and can be used for the same purpose as the guidelines. In addition, several new serum biomarker (blood) tests (for example, OVA1, Vermillion, Austin, Texas; and ROMA, Abbott Diagnostics, Lake Forest, Illinois) have recently been developed to assist the general gynecologist in deciding whether an adnexal mass is at a high enough risk of being ovarian cancer to refer the patient to a gynecologic oncologist.

When imaging tests such as ultrasound, CT scan, MRI (magnetic resonance imaging), or diagnostic laparoscopy are suspicious for ovarian cancer, then surgery is nearly always performed to obtain a definitive diagnosis, assess the nature (extent) of the cancer, and treat the disease. To assess the nature of the cancer, the surgeons stage the disease. *Staging* is the process of determining the stage of the tumor, which is determined by the location of the cancer, the size of the tumor, whether other parts of the body are affected, and the prognosis. The doctor can prescribe appropriate treatment once she or he knows the stage of the tumor. Ideally, a woman will only have to undergo one surgical procedure that will simultaneously establish the diagnosis (of ovarian cancer), determine the precise stage of disease, and remove the tumor and cancerous tissue if possible. This is one of the reasons that appropriate and accurate referral to a specialist (gynecologic oncologist) is so important. Gynecologic oncologists are trained to not only perform the diagnostic portion of the procedure (removal of the ovary) but also do a comprehensive staging procedure or debulking operation, if needed. Every woman diagnosed with an adnexal mass should feel comfortable having a conversation with her gynecologist about the level of suspicion for ovarian cancer (high or low) based on the diagnostic tests described above and about the possible need for referral to a specialist.

The symptoms of ovarian cancer can be nonspecific. In other words, as mentioned above, ovarian cancer shares many of the same presenting symptoms as other disease processes. Since those other diseases would require a different form of treatment, they must be identified or ruled out before a woman undergoes surgery for ovarian cancer. For example, the intestinal symptoms associated with diverticulitis may be confused with symptoms of ovarian cancer, but if a woman has diverticulitis, surgery for ovarian cancer will not help her diverticulitis, which is actually located in the colon. A mammogram is mandatory, and any findings must be followed up by appropriate further studies or biopsies. A colonoscopy is also mandatory. Colonoscopy may identify the true source of the patient's symptoms if they are not being caused by ovarian cancer, and it may also reveal any coexisting conditions that might require additional procedures at the time of surgery for ovarian cancer (for example, colonic polyps or colon cancer).

If the patient has a history or symptoms of upper gastrointestinal tract diseases such as peptic ulcer disease, we recommend that she also have an endoscopic evaluation of the esophagus, the stomach, and the upper small bowel. Specific studies to evaluate the drainage system of the liver, the gall bladder, and the pancreas (a test called *endoscopic retrograde cholangiopancreatography*, or ERCP) can be done if the doctor thinks the results might provide valuable information.

After all of these tests have been done and before we make a decision regarding surgery, we prefer to obtain a CT scan of the abdomen and pelvis (and sometimes the chest too), if it has not previously been done. This study helps us to accomplish two goals: first, to make sure there are no other potential causes of the symptoms (for example, pancreatic cancer or cancer of the small intestine) that would either preclude or remarkably change the surgical procedure; second, to determine how extensive the surgery needs to be within the context of the patient's ability to tolerate the surgery. Some clinicians prefer to combine the CT scan with another imaging study call a PET (positron emission tomography) scan, for a combined PET/CT scan. The PET scan measures metabolic activity and can sometimes identify small areas of disease spread that do not appear on the conventional CT scan alone. Such a finding may affect surgical planning. Once all this important information has been assembled, we begin to discuss the surgery with our patient and prepare her for surgery.

Preoperative Preparation

There is a direct relationship between how healthy a person is when he or she undergoes surgery and the chance of recovering from surgery quickly and well. We think the picture of this "health" includes more than just having well-controlled diabetes or normal blood pressure. It also includes being emotionally and psychologically ready for what might happen. And the only way a person can be prepared, as the saying goes, is to be prewarned. Keeping this in mind, during the preoperative period, the surgeon and the surgical team should take as much time as is needed to educate each patient, so that she will fully understand what is going to happen and have all her questions answered. Being well informed about what is likely to happen as well as what could happen with surgery goes a long way toward minimizing the "fear factor."

Before surgery, most patients have a chest X-ray, an electrocardiogram, and an array of blood tests. (These "pre-op" tests are done in addition to the tests mentioned above.) The patient is asked to visit her primary care provider for an overall examination and to make sure that any medical problems she has are being managed and are under control, if possible. Sometimes it is necessary to do special studies (a stress test or an echocardiogram) to determine how healthy her heart is, or to do pulmonary function tests to evaluate the health of her lungs. These tests help make sure there are no unknown risks to the patient in undergoing surgery.

In most cases the patient meets with the anesthesia team, who examine her and discuss the choices for anesthesia and postoperative pain management. And of course, before surgery, insurance company approval must be obtained, or an alternative method of payment must be verified, generally with the hospital's business office.

The preoperative visit with the surgical team is very important. Generally, the patient meets with the surgical team a week or so before the surgery. During this visit, the reason for surgery as well as the risks, benefits, and other options are reviewed. The "nuts and bolts" of the surgical procedure are described step by step for the patient. In other words, the surgeon will go through every possible contingency in a stepwise fashion and will explain what will happen for every possible finding: "If we find *this*, then we will do *this*," and so on. The patient should feel free to ask questions about the different aspects of the planned procedure until she fully understands what is going to happen. It is the surgeon's responsibility to make recommendations for treatment that, according to standard medical practice, are in the best interests of the patient. However, the autonomy and wishes of the patient must always be respected as the ultimate factor that determines what and how much surgery is actually performed. Because we cannot consult with the patient herself *during* the surgery, the preop visit is our opportunity to make sure that she and we are "on the same page" about what to do for every specific operative finding. It is a good idea to bring a family member or close friend to the preoperative counseling visit as a "second set of ears" and to write any specific questions down beforehand to make sure that all of the patient's and family's concerns are addressed completely.

The evening before surgery, the patient may be asked to empty her bowel by going through a bowel preparation. Preparing the bowel for surgery usually involves a combination of taking oral cathartics (for example, magnesium citrate) and enemas. Antibiotics may also be given, to reduce the bacterial content in the colon and minimize the risk of contamination if bowel surgery is necessary. In recent years, many surgeons (including us) have moved away from universal bowel preparation for all patients and require it only for selected cases. Recent research indicates that patients tolerate surgery much better and recover more quickly if they do not undergo a bowel "prep," and in most cases, forgoing the prep does not increase the risk of complications if the surgeon needs to make an incision into the intestine or do a resection of (that is, remove) a segment of the intestine to remove all the cancer. If ovarian cancer has spread to the bowel wall, then the surgeon may need to resect the involved portion of intestine and perform a *re-anastomosis,* hooking back together the tumor-free bowel on either side of the removed portion of intestine.

Finally, the patient's nutritional state plays a major role in how she does in surgery. We are convinced of the value of preoperative nutritional support. Scientific research has shown that when a patient has had significant weight loss or is malnourished, preoperative calorie and essential element supplementation can decrease the risk of significant side effects and even death around the time of surgery. When we are first consulted by patients who have diagnostic findings suspicious for ovarian cancer, we automatically address the issue of nutrition. Occasionally we will go beyond prescribing oral supplementation (high-calorie, high-protein meal plans) to prescribe a ten-day or longer period of intravenous (IV) nutrition before surgery. Only rarely do we delay a patient's surgery to allow for the ten days of IV nutrition, although, in the patient's best interest, we have done so.

Postoperative care is described at the end of this chapter.

Surgical Consent

Signing a surgical consent is more than a necessary medical-legal formality. It is *the conclusion of a process* during which the individual who is to undergo the surgery is educated about the procedure that will be done, the goals of the surgical procedure, the alternatives to undergoing surgery, and the complications that can occur (this should include a thorough listing of both immediate and delayed complications and side effects). We strongly believe that if at all possible, the consent

- should be obtained by the senior operating surgeon;
- should be obtained a couple of days before the surgery; and
- should be obtained only after an extensive educational effort.

The consent form has two parts. The first part should describe the reason for surgery, the planned procedure, and any additional procedures that may be warranted depending on the operative findings. If the patient is not entirely comfortable with this part of the consent, she may request that modifications be made that more accurately reflect her wishes and priorities. The second part of the informed consent should review the potential risks and complications of the surgery. Signing the informed consent does not mean that all the proposed procedures will necessarily be performed, nor that all the possible complications described will occur. A patient's signature on the informed consent simply indicates that her surgeon has explained these aspects of the surgery in sufficient detail so that the patient understands and agrees to undergo the stated procedure or procedures.

If a nurse or a surgical assistant whom the patient may have never met obtains the consent early on the morning of surgery, immediately before the patient is to be taken into the operating room and while the patient is being poked and prodded in a half-naked state—this just doesn't allow the patient to make a clear-minded decision. In rare circumstances, in an acute situation, it may be necessary to obtain consent on the morning of surgery, so that the surgery can be done as soon as possible. In any case, the patient has the right to request that the senior surgeon review the above issues with her personally and to her satisfaction. Obtaining the informed consent for surgery is an essential and, in our view, nearly sacred *process.*

Fertility Preservation

Often, young women who are faced with surgery for a possible ovarian cancer are concerned about preserving their ability to conceive a child and carry the child to delivery. The patient and her surgeon need to discuss this concern before surgery. Although the most common type of ovarian cancer, epithelial carcinoma (the type that originates from the cells on the surface of the ovary), does not usually occur at an age when women want to maintain fertility, it does sometimes occur in younger women. Certain other types of ovarian cancer (those that originate from the cells that produce the eggs) most often affect young women in their late teens. So, for many women, preserving fertility is a real concern.

Among reproductive-aged women with a newly diagnosed ovarian cancer, those whose disease appears to be confined to a single ovary (Stage IA) are the best candidates for fertility-preserving surgery. The primary goals of the surgical procedure for these women are to remove all the disease that is visible to the naked eye and to perform a complete examination of the pelvis and abdomen (staging procedure) to make sure the disease has not spread beyond the involved ovary. Often these two goals can be accomplished without removing both ovaries, both fallopian tubes, and the uterus. Although a woman who has had one tube and one ovary removed has a 10 to 15 percent absolute reduction in fertility (from an 85% chance of pregnancy by the end of one year of regular unprotected sexual intercourse to a 70% chance), the likelihood of her conceiving is still very high.

In fertility-preserving surgery for ovarian cancer, only those reproductive organs that are visibly involved with the cancer should be removed, although any suspicious cysts or lumps on an otherwise normal-appearing ovary must be biopsied. Whatever reproductive organs can be left should be left because, thanks to modern assisted-reproductive technology and surrogacy, many potential combinations of organs and donors can lead to a pregnancy.

If chemotherapy is recommended for a woman who still wishes to conceive a child, it is important to do what can done to protect the unreleased eggs (the eggs that have not ovulated yet) in the remaining ovary. Unreleased eggs can usually be protected by temporarily stopping egg production (ovulation). Ovarian suppression can be accomplished in several ways. Gonadotropin-releasing hormone agonists can be used to suppress ovarian function, but because they suppress ovarian steroid hormone production as well as egg production, they are associated with menopausal-type symptoms. We prefer to use birth control pills (OCPs), which conserve egg production without causing menopausal symptoms; we start them as soon as possible after the surgery has been completed and the decision has been made for chemotherapy.

Initial Surgery

There are two essential and primary goals of initial ovarian cancer surgery. As we state several times in this chapter, these goals are most often met when the patient is cared for by an ovarian cancer specialist (gynecologic oncologist). The goals are, first, to remove all the cancer that is evident (this is called *cytoreductive*, or *debulking*, surgery) and, second, to do surgical staging. We discuss staging first and then debulking surgery. Then we turn to the other roles of surgery in managing ovarian cancer.

Staging

Ovarian cancer is a surgically staged disease (see table 2.1). This means that the stage of ovarian cancer can *only* be determined after a surgical procedure is performed, and this procedure includes taking biopsies of the sites where the disease is likely to have spread.

It is in the patient's best interest to have the surgical staging performed at the same time as the initial surgery for the management of the tumor (adnexal mass) that led to the surgery in the first place. Determining the stage of the cancer is of value both for determining treatment (specifically, whether a patient should receive chemotherapy, and if so, how much) and for predicting outcome (the likelihood that the patient will outlive her disease). The value of performing such a procedure has been repeatedly demonstrated: 30 percent of all women with ovarian cancer that is initially thought to be isolated to the ovaries are found, at the time of surgical staging, to have cancer in sites in addition to the ovaries. Three-quarters of these women have Stage III disease.

A question that is commonly asked is whether the surgical staging procedure can be completed using a minimally invasive approach (minimally invasive surgery, or MIS), such as laparoscopy or robotic-assisted laparoscopy. The answer is that, in the hands of a skilled laparoscopic gynecologic oncologist, it *can* be done. Perhaps a more important question, however, is whether it *should* be done that way. One of the concerns, and a great source of controversy among gynecologic surgeons, is whether rupturing an ovarian cancer that appears

TABLE 2.1 *International Federation of Gynecology and Obstetrics (FIGO) Staging of Ovarian Cancer (revised January 1, 2014)*

Stage I Disease confined to one or both ovaries
    Stage IA Disease confined to one ovary
    Stage IB Disease confined to both ovaries
    Stage IC Disease confined to one or both ovaries with surgical spill of an ovarian cyst (IC1), cyst capsule rupture before surgery or cancer cells on the surface of the ovary (IC2), or cancer cells in ascites fluid or peritoneal washings (IC3)

Stage II Disease confined to the pelvis (below the pelvic brim)
    Stage IIA Disease involving the fallopian tubes and/or the uterus
    Stage IIB Disease involving other pelvic structures such as the pelvic colon, the bladder surface, or the pelvic peritoneum

Stage III Disease involving one or both ovaries with pathologically confirmed spread to the abdomen (peritoneum, organs) or retroperitoneal lymph nodes
    Stage IIIA1 Disease involving only retroperitoneal lymph nodes
    Stage IIIA2 Microscopic abdominal peritoneal involvement with or without positive retroperitoneal lymph nodes
    Stage IIIB Macroscopic (visible) abdominal peritoneal involvement less than or equal to 2cm with or without positive retroperitoneal lymph nodes; includes extension to capsule of liver or spleen
    Stage IIIC Macroscopic (visible) abdominal peritoneal involvement larger than 2cm with or without positive retroperitoneal lymph nodes; includes extension to capsule of liver or spleen

Stage IV Disease outside the abdomen (for example, in the lung or in the fluid around the lung) or involving the internal portion of the liver or spleen (parenchyma)
    Stage IVA Pleural effusion (fluid around the lung) with cancer cells in the fluid
    Stage IVB Disease involving the parenchyma of the liver or spleen; spread to organs or lymph nodes (e.g., groin) outside of the abdominal cavity

to be isolated to the ovary—a risk during MIS—has a negative effect on cure. A second concern is whether there is an increased chance of "seeding" cancer cells into the tissue where the laparoscopic port sites have been placed. We believe that, when dealing with a disease as aggressive as ovarian cancer, it is better to err on the side of being conservative. If there is any concern whether a mass is malignant (based on the presurgery imaging and blood work), we will do what we can to ensure that the mass is removed without rupture. If a colleague requests a consultation during a laparoscopic procedure on a patient who, after the ovary is removed, is diagnosed with an ovarian malignancy, we will decide whether we can perform the staging procedure using MIS.

This decision is based on numerous variables, including the patient's overall health, previous surgeries, other ongoing medical problems, and so on. It is a highly individualized decision and one that we try to avoid making without first having a thorough discussion with the patient. One way to avoid this situation is for health care providers who are not gynecologic oncologists to refer their patients to a gynecologic oncologist *before surgery* when they have any concern that an underlying ovarian cancer might exist. Excellent quality data show that a woman's chances of having the correct staging procedure performed at the time of diagnosis of her ovarian cancer are four to five times better if the operating surgeon is a gynecologic oncologist than if the surgeon is either a general surgeon or a gynecologic surgeon.

Cytoreductive Surgery

Cytoreductive surgery, or debulking, consists of removing as much of the tumor that has spread beyond the ovary as possible (removing "bulky" tumor, hence de-bulking). This type of surgery is generally a major operation, performed through a vertical midline incision in the abdomen. In most cases, the cancerous tissue beyond the ovaries is visible to the naked eye, and the goal is to remove as much of this visible disease as is safe and technically feasible.

It is not a new belief that the amount of cancer that remains after the initial surgery is directly related to the probability that a woman will survive her ovarian cancer. In fact, the first articles establishing this outcome were published when the authors of this book were still in high school and junior high! Over the intervening almost four decades, however, the medical community has learned more about the relationship between cancer remaining after surgery and survival.

Historically, the term *optimal cytoreductive* surgery indicated that *all individual tumor nodules larger than 1 centimeter* were removed. When *all visible tumor* is successfully removed, the surgery has historically been referred to as *complete cytoreduction*. As more and more scientific data accumulate, it has become clear that the greatest survival benefit is achieved when all visible disease is removed (this is termed *complete gross resection*). In fact, recent research has shown that when patients with Stage III ovarian cancer undergo a complete cytoreduction surgery with a gynecologic oncologist and are treated with intraperitoneal chemotherapy (into the abdominal cavity), 50 percent of patients survive more than ten years. Advances in surgical techniques and improvements in postoperative care have made complete cytoreduction for advanced ovarian cancer achievable in a high percentage of patients when they are cared for in a hospital with a lot of experience treating this disease. Because this is such an important issue, patients should feel empowered to talk with their surgeon beforehand about the surgeon's particular experience level with ovarian cancer and the hospital's surgical success rates.

Evidence from high-quality scientific studies increasingly supports the notion that there is absolutely nothing more important that the doctor can do to influence a woman's chance of surviving her ovarian cancer than the quality of her initial surgery and the choice of chemotherapy (the drugs and how they are administered). If a gynecologic oncologist is the primary operating surgeon, the chance that a woman will have the best surgery possible (optimal or complete cytoreduction) is three times higher than if a surgeon who is not a gynecologic oncologist performs the surgery. Sadly, however, only between 30 and 50 percent of the women with ovarian cancer in any given geographic region will have optimal surgery. Data such as these make us plead with our nongynecologic oncology colleagues to refer any of their patients who have a significant chance of having an ovarian cancer to one of the over one thousand gynecologic oncologists in the United States.

What is it about debulking surgery to remove large amounts of cancer that has such a remarkable effect on the chances that a woman will survive? It appears that multiple processes are involved. First, when the large volume of tumor has been removed, the patient is healthier overall, because she no longer has to "feed" the cancer.

Feeding the cancer drains calories and other essential nutrients from her vital organs. She will also feel better, because she will no longer have the pressure and other *mass effects* of the tumors. Mass effects are the symptoms caused by a large ovarian tumor mass pressing on nearby organs, such as the bladder or the intestine. These may include urinary frequency or constipation, for example.

Second, it appears that when all large tumor implants are removed, any residual cancer cells are more likely to be killed by the chemotherapy that follows surgery. This improved chance of killing the cells is thought to be a result of three things:

1 The remaining cancer cells grow more rapidly in response to removal of the large tumors. Because growing cancer cells are the only cells that can be killed by chemotherapy, this growth makes the remaining cells susceptible to chemotherapy.

2 The blood flow to the site of the cancer cells improves, which makes it easier to get both immune cells and anticancer drugs to the location where they are most needed.

3 Larger tumors are also more likely to contain cancer cells that have mutated to become insensitive to the killing effects of chemotherapy. It is thought that debulking surgery, by removing these drug-resistant cancer cells, can improve the effectiveness of chemotherapy.

Because the removal of any and all evident ovarian cancer is so important in a woman's odds of survival, it is equally important to do whatever is necessary, within reason, to achieve an optimal or a complete cytoreductive surgical result. This often includes removing (in addition to the ovaries) the fallopian tubes and the uterus, a segment of the sigmoid colon and rectum, and parts of the large intestine and the small intestine. Thanks to advancements in surgical techniques and tools, *colostomy* (having the intestine drain into a bag outside the abdominal wall) is rarely necessary. The appendix, if it is present, is almost always removed.

Ovarian cancer commonly spreads to the *omentum,* an "apron" of fat hanging off the middle section of the large intestine (that is, the transverse colon). The omentum is frequently removed in its entirety to ensure removal of the maximal amount of cancer cells. Ovarian cancer can also spread to the peritoneal (or lining) surfaces of the abdomen and pelvis. Not uncommonly, a procedure termed *peritoneal stripping* will be performed, again to ensure removal of as many cancer cells as possible. Peritoneal stripping may be performed in the pelvis or the abdomen or both and is much like peeling the skin off an onion: only the outer surface lining is removed. Sometimes this procedure includes removing part of the top of the bladder.

Ovarian cancer also has a tendency to spread to the under-surface of the right side of the diaphragm, the muscle that separates the abdominal cavity (*peritoneal cavity*) from the chest (*pleural cavity*). Any tumor nodules on the diaphragm should be either excised (cut out) or destroyed using one of various special instruments. In some cases, an instrument called the *argon beam coagulator* (ABC) can be used to vaporize the implanted nodules. Sometimes, however, it is necessary to excise part of the diaphragm to remove all of the tumor. This can usually be accomplished without an additional incision beyond the one that is already made on the abdomen. In select situations, it is worthwhile to perform a *thoracoscopy* (placing a telescope through the diaphragm muscle and taking a look inside the chest) to make sure there are not any tumor nodules in the chest that need to be destroyed. Additional organs (gall bladder, spleen, liver, stomach) may also need to be removed in part or whole to successfully debulk a patient. If this is necessary, as long as it doesn't harm the patient, it should be done and usually involves a stay in the intensive care unit, or ICU. If a patient is able to undergo an optimal or a complete debulking and is a candidate for intraperitoneal chemotherapy (ideally this possibility is discussed with the surgeon during the preoperative visit), the surgeon may also place a special type of catheter (called an intraperitoneal port) within the abdominal cavity to deliver these treatments. The intraperitoneal port can be placed either at the time of the initial surgery (debulking) or at a later time, after the patient has recovered from debulking, using an MIS approach. The intraperitoneal port is ultimately removed after the treatments are completed (usually about six months later).

An emerging treatment takes the concept of regional therapy

(intraperitoneal chemotherapy) one step further and delivers a chemotherapy solution directly into the abdomen at the time of surgery, immediately following the debulking procedure. In some cases, this treatment may be combined with hyperthermia (heat), which is also directly toxic to cancer cells. This treatment is called HIPEC (for hyperthermic intraperitoneal chemotherapy) and involves a 30- to 90-minute perfusion of heated chemotherapy solution around the abdomen. Although the early reports of HIPEC appear promising, more data are needed before we know exactly which patients it will benefit the most.

Neo-adjuvant Chemotherapy and Interval Debulking Surgery

Although "up-front" (that is, before chemotherapy) debulking surgery is the gold standard treatment for ovarian cancer, there are times when performing surgery prior to chemotherapy is not in the patient's best interest. Ten to 15 percent of all women with advanced ovarian cancer are too sick to tolerate an aggressive surgery, or surgical removal is considered unsafe because imaging studies have shown their disease to be quite advanced or to be located in places that make surgical removal unsafe. Not uncommonly, we will start the surgery with laparoscopy to "take a look around" the abdomen and pelvis and determine if the disease appears resectable. If it is, then we proceed to open the abdomen through a laparotomy incision and do the debulking. If we find that the disease cannot be safely removed or that removal of the disease would require such an extensive procedure that it would significantly compromise the patient's quality of life (such as removing all or most of the intestines), we obtain enough tissue for a diagnosis and stop the procedure at that point, deferring definitive surgery to a later time. Patients like this are probably best treated with what is called *neo-adjuvant chemotherapy with interval debulking surgery.*

In *neo-adjuvant chemotherapy,* an initial chemotherapy program is administered before attempting debulking surgery (rather than afterward). The term *interval debulking* refers to the fact that the cytoreductive surgery takes place after an interval of initial chemotherapy.

If the treatment plan involves neo-adjuvant chemotherapy with interval debulking, and a diagnostic laparoscopy has not been done, the first step is to collect a small amount of tissue, either through a needle or with a small incision (usually done by ultrasound or CT guidance by an interventional radiologist), to confirm that the woman has ovarian cancer. If ovarian cancer is confirmed, then the patient receives about three cycles of standard chemotherapy (described in chapter 3). During the two to three months of chemotherapy, aggressive attempts are undertaken to make the patient as strong as possible, using nutritional support to build her strength as well as medical therapy to treat any diseases she may have, such as hypertension, diabetes, or heart disease.

After she has had the three cycles of chemotherapy, the patient will have a repeat battery of imaging studies and blood tests. If the results demonstrate that there has been a good response to the chemotherapy, and if the patient is deemed healthy enough to tolerate an attempt at interval debulking, then surgery will be undertaken. The goals at the time of interval debulking are the same as the goals of debulking surgery as described above.

Scientists believe it is important to remove all the grossly evident cancer early in the chemotherapy treatment regimen to avoid having the patient develop *chemotherapy drug resistance*. In chemotherapy drug resistance, the cancer cells, being very adaptive, develop ways (often by mutating) to resist the killing effects of the chemotherapy. It has been proved that the more cancer cells there are, the larger the tumor nodules are; and the more cycles of chemotherapy that have been administered, the greater the chance of drug resistance. In neo-adjuvant chemotherapy with interval debulking, a race takes place between, on the one hand, getting the patient healthy enough for surgery and getting the tumors small enough that they can be safely removed, and on the other, the cancer cells' ability to develop a way to resist the chemotherapy agents. No one knows exactly the ideal time for interval cytoreduction in order to have the best chance of winning this race, or to achieve "the perfect balance," but the best time for most patients seems to be after three to four cycles of chemotherapy.

Secondary Debulking

If the disease comes back, additional surgery may or may not be an option. It depends on how long the disease has been gone and in how many places it has reappeared. The concept of operating again on women who have recurrent ovarian cancer is called *secondary debulking,* or *secondary cytoreductive surgery.* As the name implies, the surgeon is attempting for the second (or third or fourth) time to remove the cancer. More information is available all the time to help doctors determine who might benefit from such an attempt. The concept of secondary debulking is controversial, however, and recommendations regarding its use may vary from hospital to hospital and from surgeon to surgeon.

This type of procedure is often more difficult and riskier than the initial surgery, primarily for these three reasons:

1 Scarring from the initial surgery makes the surgery more difficult for both surgeon and patient.
2 The recurrent disease may be more deeply embedded in tissues than the earlier tumors were.
3 The patient may not be as physically fit as she was at the time of the initial debulking.

Between 12 and 25 percent of women who have secondary (or tertiary, and so forth) debulking surgery suffer a potentially life-threatening complication. Because of the very real risk of such a complication, we must be able to predict as accurately as possible before surgery which patients are going to benefit from the operation. We use a few general criteria. The women who are more likely to benefit from secondary debulking than to suffer a complication from it are women who

- have had a relatively long disease-free period (at least six months, but the longer the period, the better);
- have physical and radiographic findings that show an isolated, solitary lesion or two (three lesions at most); and
- have the physical reserve and psychological strength to undergo further chemotherapy.

The procedure is not without risk. Recurrent ovarian cancer commonly involves the intestine, and a portion of the intestine may need to be removed (and the tumor-free ends reattached) in the course of secondary debulking. Because of the complexity of these operations, blood loss can occur, and a transfusion may be necessary. In addition, healing of the wound is often complicated by infection, separation, or hernia. Some degree of bowel dysfunction is also common. This may take the form of

- *ileus,* a slow return of normal bowel function as a result of literally slow bowel (which is usually managed by resting the bowel—taking nothing by mouth—until the bowel has a chance to recover);
- *bowel obstruction,* a blockage of the flow of fluid and food through the bowel (a partial bowel obstruction may respond without surgery to a course of bowel rest with a draining tube through the nose or the abdominal wall into the stomach, along with fluids, antibiotics, and nutritional support, or it may require surgical correction—but see below); or
- *fistula,* in which a hole develops between the intestine and the abdominal or vaginal wall and fluid from inside the intestine drains out. (Fistulas sometimes heal spontaneously but may require additional surgery to repair the leak.)

Women who have a successful secondary debulking (that is, one that is "complete" as described earlier in this chapter) will have about twice the life expectancy of women who either do not undergo the debulking or who do not have a successful procedure. This is why we strongly encourage our patients who are candidates for this treatment option to consider having this surgery.

Palliative Surgery

When ovarian cancer returns and is no longer responsive to further therapy, medical problems such as bowel obstruction often develop. These problems theoretically could be treated surgically. It has been shown, however, that with rare exceptions, under these circumstances the surgery is more likely to harm the woman than to eliminate the symptoms. Similarly, we know that trying to surgically repair a bowel obstruction when the end of life is near is more likely to shorten a woman's life than to alleviate her suffering and prolong a meaningful existence.

One procedure that is often performed to improve the quality of life for women who have nausea and vomiting because of bowel obstruction is the placement of a *percutaneous gastrostomy* (PEG) tube. If the nausea and vomiting cannot be controlled with antinausea medications and IV fluids, then a PEG is placed in the woman's stomach by endoscopy. In this procedure, a long, thin tube is slipped into the stomach through the mouth.

A PEG tube, which drains the stomach directly through the anterior (front) abdominal wall, can significantly improve comfort. It allows the stomach and intestines to be drained, acting as an "overflow valve"; furthermore, there is no need for the patient to have a fixed tube between her stomach and her nose, and she will not have to vomit. The PEG also allows her to take in fluids—an action that we have found can be remarkably emotionally gratifying and physically satisfying for patients—without the fear that she will vomit the fluids back up in a few minutes. In some cases, a bowel obstruction may be due to blockage of the lower colon from progressive ovarian cancer in the pelvis. If the disease is not able to be surgically resected or treated effectively with more chemotherapy, a colostomy may be an option to relieve the bowel blockage and improve quality of life and comfort level. This is a very personal decision, and the option of colostomy surgical management should be discussed thoroughly by the patient and her doctors.

Postoperative Care

There is a dominant view—in our opinion incorrect—that to maximize healing and recovery, the postoperative patient should physically do as little as possible. Nothing could be further from the truth. We know that the sooner women become active, the less likely they are to suffer surgical side effects.

Surgical side effects include

- infections
- blood clots in the large vessels in the legs or pelvis—and pulmonary emboli, which occur when the clots break off and go to the lungs
- bowel dysfunction (ileus)
- muscle loss and weakness

There is a lot of truth to the saying "Use it or lose it," particularly when it has to do with muscle function and strength. We recommend that patients get up and out of bed as soon after surgery as they can. Of course, as our patients are finding their "land legs," it is important for someone to help them get in and out of the bed or chair and to serve as a support, if necessary, when they are walking. When patients go home, we allow them to do light lifting (less than 25 pounds), walk up and down stairs, get out to the store or religious services, and go on short car or train rides.

Another inappropriate limitation, in our view, is the prohibition on showering and getting the wound wet. As with walking around, there needs to be someone on hand to help and offer support, as a precaution against falling. But there is little chance of harm coming to a patient by getting the wound wet. Remember, the body is 75 percent water, and it is water that is helping the healing process. Getting an incision wet, or an IV or central line wet, has never to our knowledge been shown to have any negative effect on healing. The wound itself is "closed" by 18 to 24 hours after the stitches or staples have been placed. For this reason, although the wound has many months to go before the area regains its maximal strength, it would be difficult to harm it just by letting warm, soapy water rinse over it. And oh, how wonderful it feels to be clean after a couple of days in bed!

As you can see, we are generally liberal about what we allow our patients to do. We encourage them to be reasonable about driving after surgery, however. Just as it is against the law to drive with a blood alcohol level of 0.08 percent, it is also against the law to drive with narcotic pain medications circulating in the bloodstream. Beyond the slowed reaction time and impaired judgment, what about the ability to quickly move that foot from the gas to the brake when a buffoon runs the stoplight in front of you? De-acceleration injuries like those that occur in automobile accidents can damage abdominal wall wounds and lead to hernias in the incision. Therefore, we want our patients to wait to drive until they are off narcotic pain medications and can move their legs freely and without restriction when in the sitting position.

Chapter 6 of this book is devoted to the issue of nutrition. We strongly encourage the reader to take the time to go through that chapter. But several general comments about postoperative nutrition are appropriate here. For most patients, the only special recommendations we give are the following:

1 Stay well hydrated. There is a natural tendency to become dehydrated, particularly in the postoperative period. In and of itself, dehydration can lead to constipation. The rule of eight 8-ounce glasses of noncaffeinated drinks per day is a good one.

2 Avoid greasy, fatty, and spicy foods. Once a patient of ours ate a meal when she left the hospital that consisted of a raw onion salad with a spicy olive oil dressing. And she wondered why she ended up in the emergency department later that evening with a world-class upset stomach! Surgery leads to stress; this stress leads to subclinical (that which cannot be detected by a physical examination) irritation of the lining of the stomach (the gastric mucosa). That is one reason why patients are often prescribed anti-ulcer medication in the immediate postoperative period. No matter how tough one's stomach is normally, it is going to be more sensitive for a while after surgery. Be nice to it and give it soothing, relatively bland comfort foods.

3 Get lots of bulk in your diet. The intestine may have been cleaned by the preoperative bowel prep, and it probably has not had anything substantial to digest for at least several days. Now it has to be filled up again. But you want to fill it with food that is going to go through it at a fast enough pace and hold enough water so it won't bog down and you won't get constipated. Fresh fruits (nonacidic) and vegetables,

whole-grain foods, and so on are the order of the day. Avoid the so-called BRAT foods (bananas, rice [white], applesauce, and toast) that many of us have used to control diarrhea in our children.

In this chapter we have described the approach to the diagnosis of ovarian cancer, the importance of selecting the most qualified surgeon to perform the operation, and much of what a woman can expect before, during, and after surgery for ovarian cancer. After surgery, most patients begin treatment with chemotherapy. That is the focus of our next two chapters.

CHAPTER 3

Chemotherapy

Deborah K. Armstrong, MD

W hat is chemotherapy? The term means different things to different people. Literally, *chemotherapy* means using *chemicals* (chemo) as *treatment* (therapy). Whenever a chemical of any kind is used in treatment of any kind, that's chemotherapy. Treat a yeast infection with an antiyeast cream—that's chemotherapy. Take an antibiotic to treat acne—that's chemotherapy. Take hormone replacement therapy to alleviate hot flashes—that's chemotherapy. And so is taking paclitaxel (Taxol) and carboplatin as a treatment for ovarian cancer after surgery.

What we usually mean when we use the term *chemotherapy* in the context of treating ovarian cancer is the *use of drugs that are administered with the specific intent to kill cancer cells or stop cancer cell growth.* And that is how we use the term in this book. In this chapter we describe how chemotherapy is currently used in treating ovarian cancer.

Three notes before we begin. First, you may hear health care providers use the term *cytotoxic agent* when referring to chemotherapy; this generally refers to drugs that kill cancer cells. Drugs that stop cancer cell growth but don't immediately kill cells are sometimes called *cytostatic agents.* Second, many of the new drugs under investigation are cytostatic and may ultimately prove effective at preventing cancer cells from growing; some of these drugs are discussed later in this chapter. We look forward to having even more effective drugs to use in treating our patients in the future. Third, as with surgery, there are many different types of chemotherapy and different ways to administer chemotherapy for ovarian cancer. What this chapter presents is the author's philosophy on "best care" practices as they exist today. Subtle differences in the recommendations of different health care providers certainly exist; again, these are based on an individual's personal experience and on the results of ongoing research studies.

We discuss chemotherapy for epithelial ovarian cancer first. Treatments for non-epithelial cancer are discussed later in the chapter.

Optimal Chemotherapy

Although there is some controversy among experts about how to define the concept of *optimal chemotherapy* ("best chemotherapy"), nearly everyone agrees that it is a goal we should strive to reach. Simply stated, optimal chemotherapy is chemotherapy that is given at the dose that is *maximally effective* while *minimizing chemotherapy-related side effects* to avoid compromising the patient's health and general well-being. Unquestionably, this balance can be difficult to maintain.

If the scales are tipped one way or the other, it is often toward the side of maximal effectiveness, even if there is a real (but, it is hoped, transient) compromise in a patient's quality of life. Here, as with all decisions regarding ovarian cancer treatment, the woman with the disease needs to be actively involved with the decision making. Specifically, in the case of optimal chemotherapy, an individual may be willing to take the potential risk of receiving a lower, and potentially less effective, dose of chemotherapy if such a dose reduction means that the chemotherapy-related side effects are tolerable to her. Much of this chapter and all of chapter 4 focus on the prevention and control of chemotherapy-related side effects. Without these efforts to prevent and control side effects, optimal chemotherapy is very difficult to tolerate.

How Chemotherapy Works

Though it is not quite this simple, chemotherapy can be understood as working in one of two ways. Chemotherapy either (1) directly kills or accelerates the death of a cancer cell (is *cytotoxic*) or (2) prevents the cancer cell from successfully replicating or duplicating (is *cytostatic*). Most chemotherapeutic agents work against cancer through a combination of these two pathways, but one of the two pathways predominates in each agent.

To understand how chemotherapy works, we have to begin by recalling (from chapter 1) how cancer cells are different from normal cells—that is, noncancerous cells. The differences are a matter of degree, but in general the greatest difference is that cancer cells are uncontrolled in four ways: how their replication is controlled, how fast they replicate, how long they live, and where they grow.

All normal cells reproduce themselves at a rate in the healthy state that has been optimized over millions of years of evolution or as a result of divine creation (depending on one's view). They grow at just the right pace to maintain the function of the organ or group of organs they are part of. A good example of this process occurs when the skin is injured: skin grows back (through the process of cell replication) at a rapid rate until the site of injury is healed. In some situations (such as when keloids [excessive scar tissue] occur) there is exuberant growth, and the scar is thicker than necessary for the integrity of the skin. But even in these instances, the growth doesn't extend beyond where the scar should be, and it generally doesn't interfere with function.

The problem with cancer cells is that they don't stop. *They keep replicating.* Normal cells grow in a regulated way. Their growth responds to signals that tell them when to reproduce and when to stop reproducing. The regulation of cell growth is similar to the controls on a car, with a gas pedal to accelerate and a brake pedal to stop. Cancer cells have lost this regulation. Cancer cell growth becomes uncontrolled when the gas pedal is always to the floor and when the brakes aren't working. In a cell, acceleration comes from stimulating what are called *growth factor pathways*. Cancer cells can have too many growth pathways, or the pathway may be continuously in the "on" position, where it does not respond to stop signals. Similarly, cancer cells can lose the ability to stop or brake cell growth. The brakes on cell growth are called *tumor suppressors*; these suppressors are commonly lost in cancer cells.

When growth signals are not controlled, cancer cells are continuously making new *deoxyribonucleic acid* (DNA). As noted above, to stop the cancer cells, we attempt to interfere with their ability to replicate; if they cannot replicate, they die. Or else we allow them to replicate, but we cause them to live for a shorter time; they can't replicate as fast while they are dying. The latter process is called *apoptosis,* or *programmed cell death* (or *cell suicide,* referred to in chapter 1). One of the problems with cancer cells is that they live longer than normal cells; apoptosis attempts to change that situation.

The chemicals that interfere with the ability of a cell to replicate do so by interfering with the production of specific cell chemicals or structures needed for successful cell division. With regard to the chemicals that stimulate programmed cell death, scientists do not fully understand the complex process. It probably involves stimulating certain genes in the cell that were not functioning previously.

None of the chemotherapy agents we currently use are 100 percent specific in their effects. That is, these chemicals affect not only cancer cells but also normal cells. Chemotherapy produces side effects precisely because normal cells are also affected.

Chemotherapy for Epithelial Ovarian Cancer

Front-Line Chemotherapy

In any cancer treatment, front-line therapy is the first chemotherapy given. It is designed to eradicate any cancer cells remaining after surgery (if surgery has been performed) and to achieve a complete clinical remission. A *complete clinical remission* means that, after treatment, there is no evidence of detectable cancer based on physical examination, imaging studies (for example, CT scan [computed tomography] or MRI [magnetic resonance imaging]), or serum tumor markers such as CA-125. (Serum tumor markers are blood tests used to monitor the cancer, and CA-125 is a serum tumor marker used to monitor ovarian cancer.)

Front-line therapy for epithelial ovarian cancers may vary slightly from hospital to hospital, and medical center to medical center, in the United States, as well as from country to country around the world, but there is general agreement about what constitutes standard front-line therapy. The present standard is a combination of two different chemicals: a *platinum drug* (either *cisplatin* or *carboplatin*) and *paclitaxel* (Taxol). These drugs have consistently been demonstrated to be the most effective up-front combination. Medical science marches on, however, and there are ongoing investigations to determine if adding another agent with or after paclitaxel and platinum can improve either the outcome or the *toxicity profile* (the side effects).

At the Johns Hopkins Hospital and Medical Institutions, we have two preferred regimens to give after initial surgery. One is intravenous (or IV) paclitaxel and carboplatin. The other is a combination of IV and *intraperitoneal* (or IP, which means the medication is infused directly into the abdominal cavity) paclitaxel and cisplatin, also called IV/IP therapy.

Baseline tests

Before the chemotherapy is administered, we draw blood from the patient to obtain a set of baseline laboratory studies: a complete blood count (CBC) with differential and platelet count as well as a full chemistry panel. We also obtain a baseline CA-125 or other tumor-related markers and sometimes baseline imaging (usually a CT scan of the chest, abdomen, and pelvis). These studies are extremely important. We will compare them with laboratory and imaging study results during and after administration of chemotherapy to determine whether the chemotherapy is working and is being tolerated.

Central access catheter

A central access catheter has certain advantages for patients receiving chemotherapy. Most central access catheters are *semipermanent*, meaning that the catheter will stay in place for the duration of chemotherapy and will be removed afterward. A central access catheter has a real advantage because it provides a dependable infusion site for drawing blood tests and for IV administration of chemotherapy and other treatments (such as medications and blood transfusions). Placing a central catheter requires a minor (same day) surgical procedure. Some maintenance is required, such as periodic injections of heparin, a blood thinner, to keep the line open.

There are two main types of central access catheters: external and implanted ports. External catheters are just that—access ports with one end located outside of the body; these catheters eliminate the need to stick the skin each time medication is administered, blood is drawn, or the port is flushed with heparin. Because the external port lacks the protection of an overlying layer of skin, however, it must be carefully cared for each day to prevent infection. External catheters are usually inserted in the forearm (called a PICC line, for *peripherally inserted central catheter*). Less commonly, a catheter can be inserted just under the collarbone (called a Hickman catheter). Implanted ports have a reservoir that is entirely underneath the skin; they have the advantage of a lower infection risk but the disadvantage of requiring a needle stick each time the catheter is accessed for infusion.

Delivering IP chemotherapy into the peritoneal cavity requires a surgical procedure to implant an access port under the skin of the abdomen, so chemotherapy can drain directly into the abdomen and pelvis. This port is sometimes implanted at the initial debulking surgery, or it can be implanted later, before chemotherapy, as a minor (same day) surgery, sometimes using laparoscopy. This catheter is similar to (and sometimes identical to) the implanted ports used for IV access. These catheters have a reservoir that is located underneath the skin. The reservoir is easily accessed by a special needle called a Huber needle, which is inserted through the overlying skin, allowing the IP therapy to flow through a tube connected to the needle.

Chemotherapy schedule

Different chemotherapy drugs or combinations of drugs can be administered over different time intervals, in what is called the *chemotherapy schedule*. Most drugs or drug regimens used to treat ovarian cancer are given every three to four weeks. This amount of time allows the body's normal blood cells (red blood cells, white blood cells, and platelets) to recover from the effects of one treatment and be ready for the next one. For some patients, however, the drug may be administered weekly or even daily, depending on the specific drug dose and schedule. Whatever treatment interval is prescribed, it is important to try to stay on schedule as much as possible to maximize the cancer-killing ability of the chemotherapy. If the normal blood cells are slow to recover, the treatment may need to be delayed. A delay of a week or so will not have any meaningful impact on the effectiveness of chemotherapy; because of this, we will occasionally modify the treatment schedule by a week or so to allow our patients to participate in important personal, social, or professional events without having to deal with the immediate side effects of chemotherapy or other chemotherapy-related disruptions.

Our plan generally is to administer six cycles of chemotherapy. If a woman has had optimal cytoreductive surgery (see chapter 2), there is generally no disease to follow on imaging. In this case we follow the CA-125 with each cycle. If it declines or is normal, no further imaging is done during chemotherapy. For patients who had visible disease on imaging studies before chemotherapy, we will usually repeat a series of imaging studies. The purpose of the reassessment is to make sure that the cancer is responding appropriately to the chemotherapy treatment. In rare instances, the standard chemotherapy program of paclitaxel and platinum may not kill the remaining cancer cells effectively. If the imaging studies indicate that this is the case, then the treatment program may be modified by, for example, changing to a different combination of drugs. For the small percentage of women whose initial cytoreductive surgery was not optimal, we will consider another attempt at debulking surgery. The decision whether to recommend further surgery is based on these studies showing whether a patient has had an adequate response to treatment. For a woman who has not had any cytoreductive surgery and is undergoing *neo-adjuvant* chemotherapy, we will use the reassessment studies to determine whether an attempt at debulking should now be made. Neo-adjuvant chemotherapy is chemotherapy that is given before cytoreductive surgery—for instance, when there is vast disease—to attempt to shrink the cancer so that the surgical procedure is not as extensive.

The day of administration

The day of administration actually starts the night before. We recommend that our patients eat lightly the night before, choose nonspicy and nongreasy foods, and avoid heavy foods (like large portions of meat). For patients who have had difficulty with nausea during previous chemotherapy cycles, we may start antinausea medications the night before and continue them the next morning (please see table 4.5 in chapter 4). We also strongly recommend that our patients take in lots of noncaffeinated and nonalcoholic fluids (more than eight glasses in all) during the afternoon, evening, and morning before the chemotherapy. We have found over the years that a lot of the unpleasant feelings patients have the first few days after chemotherapy are due to dehydration as much as anything else. They just don't want to push anything in after a dose of chemotherapy, and therefore they naturally "prune out." Women who "supersaturate" or "tank up" as much as possible before the chemotherapy really seem to do better.

Generally, for IV chemotherapy, it takes about half a day to administer one cycle of carboplatin (carbo) and paclitaxel. After the laboratory results have been checked, the pre-chemotherapy medications have been given, and the dosing of the chemotherapy has been triple-checked, the chemicals are administered. The paclitaxel is given first, running in the line over about 3 hours. This is followed by the carboplatin, which is given over about a half hour. The paclitaxel is administered slowly to avoid an allergic reaction to either the paclitaxel or the fluid it is mixed in. If a patient has become anemic and needs a blood transfusion, we generally try to do this at the same session and will infuse the blood after the chemotherapy is "in" and we are satisfied that everything is going well.

There are three parts to IV/IP chemotherapy: IV paclitaxel given day 1, IP cisplatin given day 2, and IP paclitaxel given day 8. It is easy to see that this is a more complicated regimen than just the IV therapy. On day 1, pre-medications are given, then the IV paclitaxel is given slowly into the IV line over 3 hours, just as above. On day 2, patients will return to the infusion center. Day 2 is a longer day due to the requirements for IV fluids before and after the cisplatin. On day 2 patients will have additional pre-chemotherapy medications, then will have fluid infused through the IV and through the IP port followed by the IP cisplatin. On day 8 patients will again have pre-medications, then fluid infused through the IP port followed by IP paclitaxel.

Women who were not optimally debulked at initial surgery may have another surgery after two to four cycles of chemotherapy. This is referred to as an interval debulking surgery. For women who are optimally debulked with interval surgery, an IP port is sometimes placed, and they are switched to the IV/IP chemotherapy for the remainder of their chemotherapy treatments. Although we don't yet know if this is as good as having IV/IP therapy for all chemotherapy treatments, it gives these women the chance to have some of the benefit from IV/IP chemotherapy even if they weren't optimally debulked with the first surgery.

When her vital signs are fine and any short-term side effects cleared up, the patient is ready to go home. Several of the medications that are given before chemotherapy (for example, diphenhydramine [Benadryl] or lorazepam [Ativan]) may cause drowsiness, so we strongly recommend that a friend or a family member drive the patient home after treatment.

This is critical: all prescriptions must either be filled in the hospital pharmacy before a patient goes home from her chemotherapy infusion or be ready to be picked up on the way home. Patients should not have to go out again to get medications, a trip that is nearly impossible when you are not feeling well. Chapter 4 discusses the medications we prescribe.

After chemotherapy

The majority of women experience most of the acute side effects of chemotherapy within the first few days after receiving the cytotoxic agents. In the period immediately after treatment, usually about three to five days, some women have muscle aches and joint pains (paclitaxel in particular can cause these pains). Mild analgesics such as acetaminophen (Tylenol), naproxen (Aleve), or ibuprofen (Motrin) often provide effective relief for muscle aches. Most patients receiving chemotherapy experience some degree of fatigue after treatment. The fatigue may last from a couple of days to a week or more. This toxicity can be cumulative; in other words, the longer the treatment goes on, the more tired the patient is after each treatment. Once the entire treatment course is completed, it may take several months or more to recover fully from the effects of chemotherapy.

An unsettled stomach—but not nausea per se—affects most women in the first few days after this combination of chemotherapy. We strongly urge our patients to keep taking their prophylactic antinausea medications during this period. If a woman develops nausea or vomiting, we encourage her to take different medications, as discussed in chapter 4. For the first couple of days after treatment, meals should be light, low in fat, and bland, just like the meals the night before and during chemotherapy. Many of our patients tell us that complex carbohydrates (pasta, rice, potatoes, and bread) sit well on the stomach. We can't emphasize enough the importance of staying hydrated: drink, drink, drink! (Not alcohol or caffeine, however.) For women receiving cisplatin as part of IV/IP, we sometimes recommend that they return to the infusion center two or three days after the cisplatin to get extra IV fluids and IV nausea medications.

The neuromuscular side effects that all our patients have to a lesser or greater degree are generally the most bothersome. These side effects can be divided into those that are nonspecific (feeling tired or wiped out) and those that are specific (changes in any of the five senses, though touch, taste, and hearing are most commonly affected). We discuss these side effects in chapter 4.

The other universal side effect from the paclitaxel chemotherapy is hair loss on the head. Some women also lose their eyelashes and eyebrows. Hair loss usually starts about two or three weeks after the first paclitaxel infusion. Some women report that the hair follicles hurt as the hair is coming out, particularly women with long hair. Some women get a short haircut to "ease into" their hair loss. If you have children at home, letting them help cut your hair before the chemotherapy hair loss occurs sometimes gives them a sense of control over an otherwise frightening situation for them. Generally social workers can discuss this and other ideas further with you if you like. The hair generally starts to grow in again approximately four to six weeks after the last paclitaxel infusion, depending on how fast your hair normally grows.

Getting ready for the next cycle

One of the most remarkable advances in chemotherapy is not the new drugs we use, but our ability to minimize the possibility of serious side effects or even death from the chemotherapeutic agents. Doctors have learned how important it is to keep a close eye on a patient's blood counts and laboratory values to avoid life-threatening complications. We usually recommend that patients have blood drawn for a repeat set of tests about ten to fourteen days after the first cycle of chemotherapy. If all is well, these blood tests may not need to be repeated in the middle of the cycle again. We always repeat these same tests immediately before administering the next cycle of chemotherapy. CA-125 and any other potentially valuable tumor markers can be checked monthly, though many experts argue that they need to be done only at baseline and after the third and sixth cycles.

The day or two before (or even the day of) the next dose of chemotherapy, we meet with our patients. Often this visit takes place on the morning of a half-day chemotherapy treatment scheduled for the afternoon. We find these pre-chemotherapy visits very valuable. They give us an opportunity to ask our patients specific and focused questions, answer our patients' questions, do an interval physical examination, and write or rewrite needed prescriptions. We also like to use these moments to discuss again many of the important issues surrounding living life to the fullest during chemotherapy.

Consolidation Chemotherapy

Consolidation chemotherapy (discussed here) and *salvage chemotherapy* (discussed in the next section) are important concepts in the treatment of ovarian cancer. Chemotherapy that is given after the initial chemotherapy program has been completed, when there is no clinical evidence of disease, is called *consolidation chemotherapy*, or *maintenance chemotherapy*, and can be viewed as an "insurance policy" against the cancer's recurring. Most of the time, consolidation chemotherapy is given to women who have responded to initial chemotherapy, frequently when they are apparently free of disease (as far as can be determined by physical examination, imaging studies, and blood tests).

The theory behind consolidation chemotherapy is this: we know that more than 50 percent of women who have undergone optimal surgery and optimal chemotherapy and who have no evidence of disease will still have a recurrence. It comes back because there are hidden cancer cells that initially responded to the front-line chemotherapy but did not respond completely, probably because these cancer cells possess some degree of resistance to the chemotherapy that was first administered. The thinking goes that by administering the same drugs but by a different regimen or method, or by giving different drugs by a different method, we might be able to kill these residual cancer cells in some of the women who have so-called invisible persistent disease.

It is our obligation as doctors to tell our patients about the choices in treatment options available to them as well as the risks and benefits associated with those choices. We also believe we need to provide information to our patients about how strongly the scientific data support one choice or another. Only a small amount of data supports consolidation therapy. Consolidation treatment may delay recurrence, but usually by only a few weeks, and unfortunately, to date, no consolidation therapy has been demonstrated to improve survival. If we had consolidation treatments that gave women a significantly longer time until recurrence or that allowed women to live longer, we would recommend them. For now, until some consolidation treatment is shown to do one of those things, we feel that consolidation therapy robs women of the ability to get back to some semblance of a normal life after chemotherapy and is detrimental to quality of life (after all, consolidation therapy always carries some toxicity).

Salvage Chemotherapy

Salvage chemotherapy is quite different from consolidation chemotherapy. Salvage chemotherapy is administered either when the ovarian cancer has not gone away after treatment (the patient was never disease-free) or when there is unequivocal evidence that the cancer has now come back. We know that a cure in either of these situations is unlikely, but meaningful prolongation of a productive life for many months or years is not an unreasonable goal. These different situations generally lead to different recommendations regarding treatment.

Salvage therapy for a woman who has not responded well or at all to initial treatment

We know that these patients, in general, unfortunately have the shortest life expectancy of any of our patients. Therefore issues of quality of life and how the patient wants to spend the limited amount of life she has left are of paramount importance. We have had patients in this situation who selected one of these options: no treatment and hospice support only; aggressive second-line chemotherapy using an FDA-approved drug; treatment on a clinical trial; and alternative therapy. Individuals made their decisions based on many factors: how ill they were (the sickest women generally chose no further treatment); whether there was an upcoming event that they were willing to do anything to witness (for example, the woman who chose aggressive second-line therapy because she wanted to do whatever was possible to attend her granddaughter's wedding nine months later); whether their family and other loved ones would view no treatment as giving up; and whether, though not willing to do nothing, they were also not willing to deal with the inconvenience and toxicity of cytotoxic chemotherapy (such women chose alternative treatments).

Salvage therapy for a woman who had a complete response to the initial chemotherapy

An important question here is, how long did the complete response last? How to treat a woman when the disease comes back is directly related to how long the disease was gone. In general, the longer the disease was not evident (the *disease-free interval*), the more likely it is that we would consider surgery again and recommend administering platinum-based multidrug regimens.

Although there is no hard and fast rule, our opinion is that if a woman has been disease-free for more than a year and then the ovarian cancer returns, secondary cytoreductive surgery should be considered first, and then retreatment with carboplatin and another drug should be considered. Possible regimens include carboplatin and paclitaxel, carboplatin and pegylated liposomal doxorubicin (PLD, Doxil), carboplatin and docetaxel, or carboplatin and gemcitabine. Several factors go into deciding which regimen to use, including the convenience (or inconvenience) of the regimen, toxicities experienced in the first chemotherapy, and any significant persistent toxicity, especially neurotoxicity.

When the disease has recurred in a relatively short time (less than twelve months but more than six), we might again consider performing secondary cytoreductive surgery, but this would depend on what the scans showed and the sites of the disease.

There is no limit on how many different salvage regimens a patient can receive. But when a particular regimen has failed, it is important to reevaluate the patient's goals before another regimen is started. The cancer cells that survive chemotherapy are the "bullies," and their ability to survive prior chemotherapy regimens makes them less likely to respond to subsequent treatments. Sadly, the general rule is that the more different types of chemotherapy a patient has had, the more likely it is that she will have side effects from the chemotherapy, and the less likely it is that her ovarian cancer will respond to the treatment.

Other Chemotherapy for Epithelial Ovarian Cancer

In addition to the cytotoxic agents, other drugs are used in treating women who have ovarian cancer. Although none of these approaches to treatment are considered front-line treatments in the conventional sense, many of them are of proven benefit; some others are only of potential—and as yet unproven—benefit.

Hormonal Therapy

For years, health care professionals have known that certain types of cancers respond to hormonal treatment, even when the cancer has spread. Dr. Rick Montz distinctly remembered a case when he was a second-year medical student that demonstrated the effect of hormonal treatment. On Saturday mornings, there was an optional course on clinical disease that involved the presentation of classic examples. One Saturday the students learned about a man who had developed metastatic prostate cancer. Because testosterone (the major hormone produced by the testicles) stimulates the growth of prostate cancer, the patient had undergone an orchiectomy (surgical removal of the testicles) to stop his production of testosterone. Following that treatment, his metastatic disease shrank remarkably, and his pain was significantly relieved. Unfortunately, this response didn't last for more than a year or so, but at the time of the case presentation, he was receiving estrogen, which functionally worked as an "anti-testosterone." Again, his symptoms decreased and his lesions shrunk.

This case demonstrates a phenomenon that can occur with *hormonally responsive cancers*, such as prostate, breast, endometrial, and ovarian epithelial: if you take away the hormone that stimulates the cancer (sort of "fuel for the fire"), metastatic lesions may shrink. A similar effect can sometimes be obtained by giving an antitropic (*tropic* means "growth") hormone. In a simplified fashion, these phenomena explain why tamoxifen and anastrozole (Arimidex) work as treatment for breast cancer and why select women with metastatic endometrial cancer can gain some even long-term control of their disease with the use of progesterones (working as anti-estrogens).

The unfortunate reality is that hormonal therapy works for only a small percentage of women with ovarian cancer. Only about 7 to 10 percent of women with ovarian cancer who receive hormonal therapy will have a measurable response. *Measurable response* is by convention defined as a 50 percent shrinkage in the size of the lesion, in two dimensions, lasting at least two months. Cures have never occurred with hormonal therapy.

The explanation for such a poor response rate is that as most ovarian cancers develop, the cancer cells lose their ability to respond to hormonal signals. Two types of ovarian cancer respond better than the other types to hormonal therapy: ovarian cancer that is well differentiated (sometimes called low grade) and endometrioid ovarian cancer. Well-differentiated and endometrioid cancers are more likely to retain their ability to respond to hormonal signals and to be inhibited by the effects of hormonal therapy. Dr. Deborah Armstrong cares for a woman who is 42 and was first diagnosed with a low-grade serous ovarian cancer in her early twenties. She has never responded to chemotherapy but has had responses to a series of hormonal treatments for more than ten years.

Although the majority of ovarian cancers will not be sensitive to hormonal therapy, in certain instances we think it is rational to attempt such a therapy. For women who have recurrent disease that is shown to express *hormone receptors,* it is worthwhile to attempt hormonal therapy, in our opinion. Hormone receptors might be thought of as "docking stations" in the ovarian cancer cells; they must be present for the hormones to have any effect on the cell's growth. We can predict with a fair degree of accuracy whether a woman with ovarian cancer will respond to hormonal therapy by doing specific studies (*immunohistochemistry* staining, or IHC) on cancer tissue. These studies measure the hormone receptors in cancer cells. It is always preferable to test tissue that is obtained as recently as possible, because a cancer may over time lose its receptors. Tissue to be tested for hormone receptor expression can be obtained at the time of secondary cytoreductive surgery or through a more limited biopsy of a recurrent tumor mass.

Despite our ability to predict response to hormonal therapy, we would still attempt to treat with hormones some women whose tests have shown that the cancer appears not to express the receptors. These might be women who haven't had their hormone receptors tested, for example, or women who wish to do something to continue to treat their disease but don't want to have much in the way of side effects. These women are more likely to have more mature (well-differentiated) tumors of the endometrioid variety.

Tamoxifen or one of the aromatase inhibitors (anastrozole [Arimidex], letrozole [Femara], or exemestane [Aromasin]) is the hormonal therapy usually prescribed for ovarian cancer. Side effects may include weight gain, hot flashes, bone loss, muscle and joint aches, and blood clotting.

Targeted Biologic Therapy

Ovarian cancer cells are well-oiled machines that are programmed to grow. But like all biological "machines," they require an array of complex chemicals and mechanisms to keep them functioning. Part of the medical challenge of conquering cancer cells comes from the behavior of the cells: either they lack certain gene products to help regulate (restrain) their growth, or they produce chemicals stimulating the production of all the cellular resources the ovarian cancer cells need to continue their uninhibited growth.

It has been proposed, quite rationally, that if we could devise a way to disrupt only the chemicals that stimulate growth of the cancer cells, we could then focus our therapy directly on the cancer cells and avoid negative effects on healthy tissues. Numerous experimental efforts using this approach have been made, including inhibiting the growth of blood supply that the cancer needs (*anti-angiogenesis therapy*), stimulating the cell to undergo programmed cell death (*apoptosis*), interfering with growth signals (tyrosine kinase inhibitors [TKIs]), and others. It is vital that the readers of this guide understand two essential points. First, these are great ideas, and a large number of remarkably bright and well-funded scientists are working on them. Second, progress with these agents comes in baby steps. Nothing so far has become a magic bullet for ovarian cancer. However, given the recent successes of targeted biologic therapy in some notoriously difficult cancers such as lung cancer, renal cell cancer (kidney cancer), and melanoma, as well as the ongoing genomic revolution, it is certainly a time to be hopeful. We can report progress since the first edition of this guide and fully expect that several years from now, when a subsequent edition of this guide is published, we will have many more effective growth-inhibiting treatments to report.

Antibody Therapy

Just as cancer cells are genetically different from normal cells, cancer cells can express different *antigens* (pieces of protein on the surface of the cell or elsewhere) than do noncancer cells. *Antibodies* are proteins that circulate in the blood system and react with (or bind to) antigens. Antibodies are very specific in their ability to recognize a particular antigen, sort of like being able to identify one of your family members within the multitude of people attending a rock concert. If a cell produces an antigen, then, in theory at least, science can produce an antibody against that antigen. When the antigen and the antibody bind together, they form a complex that is recognized by the body's own hunter-killer cells (the white blood cells called lymphocytes). The lymphocytes kill the cells, and the dead cells are cleared from the body by one of the body's "garbage disposal systems" (the liver is cleared via bile into the gastrointestinal tract, the kidney via the urine).

The problem with antibody therapy is that it will only work if the cell we want to kill produces a unique antigen that isn't found on the surface of normal cells. That is, we want to target the cancer cell but not the normal cell. And unfortunately, cancer cells and normal cells often produce the same antigens. To date, cancer-specific antigens have been elusive. Cancer cells do produce select antigens in higher concentrations than normal cells, however (for example, the antigen HER2/neu and the p-53 antigens). If we administer an antibody against these antigens, all cells that have the antigens will be affected, but the cancer cells more than others and, it is hoped, to such an extent that they will be killed. Because other, noncancer cells also produce the antigens, some normal, noncancerous cells will be attacked as well. It is this targeting of normal cells that leads to the side effects of antibody therapy.

In addition to being used to stimulate the immune system, antibody therapy can be used in other ways. Bevacizumab (Avastin) is an antibody to a growth factor called *vascular endothelial growth factor* (VEGF). VEGF stimulates new blood vessel formation. Cancer cells need to develop new blood vessels in order to grow, and therefore blocking new blood vessel formation has potential for anticancer therapy. In fact, bevacizumab is highly active in treating recurrent ovarian cancer. Antibodies can also be used to more specifically deliver chemotherapy to cancer cells. An antibody to HER2/neu (trastuzumab) has been linked to a potent chemotherapeutic agent (emtansine) in what is called an *antibody drug conjugate*. This drug (TDM-1 [Kadcyla]) is very effective in treating HER2/neu overexpressing breast cancer. Antibody drug conjugates are currently being tested in ovarian cancer. Another way antibodies work is by blocking growth factor receptors on the surface of cells. Antibodies such as trastuzumab and pertuzumab (Perjeta), which block activation of HER2/neu, and antibodies to other members of the epidermal growth factor receptors (EGFRs) are in common use. The idea of anticancer-specific antibody therapy makes good sense, but to date, the successes have been limited in ovarian cancer. We hope that as we learn more about what makes cancer cells different from normal cells, we will be able to find cancer-specific antigens that will allow antibody production and avoid systemic side effects.

Immunotherapy

There are differences of opinion in our understanding today of how the immune system interacts with cancer. Some experts view cancer as a failure of the immune system to recognize cells that have become "foreign," while others view cancer cells as variants (albeit vicious ones) of normal cells. When the body recognizes its own cells as foreign, the result is severe autoimmune diseases like lupus and rheumatoid arthritis. Normally, immune responses are controlled by a delicate balance between immune-stimulating cells and immune-suppressing cells. Recently, treatments such as ipilimumab (Yervoy), which interfere with immune-suppressing cells, have had amazing success in treating melanoma and other diseases. In ovarian cancer, we know that patients who have abundant immune cells (called *tumor-infiltrating lymphocytes,* or TILs) infiltrating their tumors have a better outcome with their ovarian cancer. For this reason, ovarian cancer may be a good immunotherapy target, and a number of trials are currently going on. Immunotherapy, unlike chemotherapy, which only works while it is in the body, has the potential to keep working for a lifetime if the immune cells can be "reprogrammed" to recognize the cancer cells as foreign.

Non-Epithelial Ovarian Cancers

For the most part in this chapter, we have been addressing the use of chemotherapy in the management of epithelial ovarian cancers. There are numerous reasons for this focus. First, the epithelial cancers are by far the most common. Second, treatment of these cancers is relatively similar (front-line therapy with paclitaxel and a platinum drug). Third, many of the non-epithelial cancers (the *stromal tumors*, in particular) are not as responsive to chemotherapy and therefore are not as routinely treated with a standard regimen.

Even though the stromal tumors are not responsive, the ovarian cancers called *germ cell tumors*, which arise from the cells that are part of what is needed to develop the egg, are often exquisitely responsive to multiagent chemotherapy. The ability to treat germ cell tumors has been a great advance over the last couple of decades. The germ cell malignancies are much more common in young women, who may wish to maintain their potential for childbearing. In the past, the most common germ cell malignancy, dysgerminoma, generally was treated with radiation therapy. The radiation treatment was often successful but at a cost: infertility. In contrast, multiagent chemotherapy, though it has a potentially negative effect on fertility, does not always cause infertility. When investigations in the 1980s demonstrated that we could treat these tumors with the same degree of success by using multiagent chemotherapy, a major step forward was taken in balancing treatment, on the one hand, and quality of life, on the other.

Investigational Drugs and Clinical Trials

A large percentage of women who develop ovarian cancer will have recurrence of the disease following the appropriate aggressive initial treatments. Unfortunately, it is not likely that their cancer will be responsive to approved therapies. If they wish to undergo further attempts to control their cancer, they have available to them three general options: take treatments (usually chemotherapy) that are FDA approved but not approved as treatment for ovarian cancer; take substances (whether identified as medications or in other categories, such as *herbal therapies*) that have not been proved (using traditional scientific standards for proof) to work for any cancer; or participate in an investigational trial (also called a clinical trial). It is this third alternative that we discuss in this section.

Each week we see women who have run out of approved options as treatment for their repeatedly recurrent ovarian cancer. Many of these women are looking for and willing to try nearly anything that has any real chance of meaningfully prolonging a functional life. We are impressed by how much information they possess and how deep their understanding of clinical trials often is.

Clinical trials are designed to determine, in a stepwise fashion, whether a potential treatment is as safe as, as effective as, and "as good as or better than" previously approved therapies. The steps, commonly called *phases*, are used to describe what sort of study is being conducted and what the goals of that study are.

Phase I Trials

The purpose of a phase I trial is to determine the safe and tolerable dose and schedule of any particular treatment. Phase I trials are also commonly called *dose-finding trials, toxicity trials,* or *side-effect trials.* Although data about whether the treatment works will be collected, this is not the purpose of the study. Many, many treatments are investigated in phase I trials, and some are shown to be so toxic that no further investigation is undertaken. Phase I trials sometimes allow patients with any disease to participate, but sometimes they are limited to specific diseases. This is particularly true if the agent being tested is a targeted drug that seems to make sense for those diseases. Although phase I trials might sound scary, it helps to recognize that every drug used to treat ovarian cancer went through a phase I trial. It is through these trials that we figure out how to use new drugs.

Phase II Trials

The purpose of a phase II trial is to determine whether a treatment works for a specific disease. There will sometimes be a randomized assignment of patients to either a standard treatment or the investigational agent. Sometimes the trial is done using just the investigational agent simply to answer the question, does the cancer respond? Yes or no? In the latter case, the response rates will be compared to the results of previous studies (referred to as *historical controls*). The investigating scientists will compare how many people treated with the phase II drug responded and how that response rate compares to historical information published about similar groups of individuals receiving different treatments.

Studies often combine a phase I trial and a phase II trial in an attempt to economize. Although such a combined study does not, strictly speaking, follow the rules, it makes it possible for investigators to find out more rapidly whether a drug should be quickly brought into the front line of therapy.

Phase III Trials

Phase III clinical trials are considered to be the gold standard of investigation. (The gold standard is that level of scientific evidence against which all other studies are compared.) In these trials, different people who are identified as having the same disease are treated with different therapies. Patients are assigned randomly to different therapies. This means that after the person has agreed to participate in the trial, neither the investigator nor the patient-subject has any influence over which treatment the patient receives. Usually one of the treatments used is the current standard—that is, the treatment that has proved to be the best therapy for the disease.

When no standard therapy has been identified for the specific disease, then phase III trials may compare two or more nonstandard drugs. An example of this was the trial comparing pegylated liposomal doxorubicin (Doxil) and topotecan in women whose ovarian cancer had failed to respond to both paclitaxel and the platinum drugs. For women in this situation, there is no standard therapy, but there are many different choices. The goal of the Doxil-topotecan trial was to assess both response to and toxicity of the two drugs.

The phase III trial is also called a *randomized controlled trial* (RCT). Some individuals add the term *prospective* (*prospective randomized con-*

trolled trial), implying that the trial is done in a forward data-collecting fashion. In other words, the data (for example, the likelihood of responding to treatment) are collected as the study happens in real time. In contrast, a retrospective study looks backward to collect the data (after all the responses have occurred). Scientifically speaking, the quality of information provided by prospective studies is considered superior to that of retrospective studies. This is why phase III RCTs are considered the gold standard for determining the most appropriate treatment for a particular disease.

Phase IV Trials

Phase IV clinical trials are not part of the conventional trial schedule used by the National Cancer Institute (NCI) and other government and nonprofit funding agencies. These trials, which are commonly performed and underwritten by for-profit pharmaceutical companies, are essentially investigations carried out *after* a treatment has been approved and has been demonstrated to be superior. Generally, phase IV trials are performed in an attempt to obtain more information about effectiveness and toxicity in a broader range of the population. The phase IV trial holds little unseen risk or unproven benefit for the enrollee.

Enrolling in Clinical Trials

To participate in a clinical trial, a patient has to meet a strict set of qualifications, or inclusion criteria. These criteria usually have to do with the patient's performance status (overall health), disease status (initial diagnosis or recurrence), whether there is disease that can be measured (to accurately evaluate the effectiveness of the new treatment), and the number of previous treatments the patient has received. These strict inclusion criteria are set forth to make sure all patients in a specific trial are as similar as possible, so that any improvement in outcome (that is, response) can be confidently attributed to the new treatment rather than to differences in the clinical characteristics of the individual patients.

Informed consent is a critical aspect of participating in clinical trials. Informed consent includes a discussion of the possible benefits of therapy, although in many cases, these benefits will not be precisely known (getting information about the benefits is the reason for doing the trial in the first place!). A review of the possible side effects is also included in the informed consent, and again, these may not be precisely known. For example, one of the main objectives of a phase I trial is to determine the specific side effects of a new treatment when it is given at different doses.

Response Standards in Investigational Trials

We believe it is critical for a woman and those who care about her to understand what sort of responses are being looked for in the clinical trial setting. For a person who is participating in a trial that requires measurable disease for participation, the changes in the tumor with treatment will be followed closely. There is an agreed-on way of measuring changes in tumor size called RECIST (Response Evaluation Criteria in Solid Tumors). RECIST will use the sum of the largest cross-section diameter of five to ten lesions. Disease that grows or develops new lesions is considered progression. In addition to changes in tumor size, most trials measure the time to progression (TTP), or progression-free survival (PFS). This second measurement makes it possible to measure a benefit from treatments that don't produce shrinkage but that delay tumor growth. A study might be reported as "positive" if the median PFS (the time at which half of the patients had progressed) went from six months with the standard treatment to eight months with the trial treatment. Whether two months is meaningful will depend on what the patient does during that time, feels like during that time, and anticipates after the two months are up. For example, when Dr. Rick Montz wrote the first version of this book, he had been alive 46 years or, said another way, 552 months. Two months is less than half of 1 percent of the time he had been alive. Over those two months, however, he watched his second son's varsity football team make it to the regional semifinal playoffs, saw his daughter play soccer (very well), played air guitar to a Linkin Park song with his third son while driving home from Mass with the top down on his car, watched his eldest son mature as a freshman at

Brown, was emotionally and physically intimate with his life mate, Kate, published a couple of articles, operated a bunch, consulted on scores of patients with gynecologic cancers, spent a few days in Italia with his mom and dad, and so on. We hope the point is made: though two months isn't long as a percentage of a person's life, man oh man, you can have a lot of joy in sixty days.

Whether the investment in inconvenience and side effects is worth the potential for a two-month or longer prolongation of life is an extremely personal decision. Our goal is to make sure that our patients understand what's involved when they are making decisions about treatment. It is our patients' decision whether to participate.

Finally, most trials will also follow patients for overall survival (OS), even if they are off the study and getting other treatments.

For phase I trials, response rates are not the outcomes of interest—side effects and tolerability of the treatment are. In phase III trials, response rates, PFS, and OS are compared directly to the effectiveness of the standard or comparison treatment, so the response rate of the investigational treatment is interpreted within the context of the response rate of the standard therapy being evaluated simultaneously. For example, if the investigational treatment produced a response rate of just 12 percent, this might not seem like much, but if the response rate of the standard treatment was only 6 percent, the investigational therapy would have produced a 100 percent increase in response.

Why Are Certain Treatments Never Studied?

There are many reasons some treatments are never investigated in a phase I, II, III, or IV format: first, there may be no data from nonhuman trials to indicate that the treatment may work in humans; second, there may be data from nonhuman trials to indicate that the treatment may work in humans, but the trials may have also shown so much toxicity that humans clearly could not take the treatment; and finally, it may be that no one is willing to pay for the study.

It happens often that no one is willing to pay for a study, and this phenomenon has little to do with science and everything to do with the business of medicine. If there is no profit to be made once the treatment is proved to work, no for-profit company is going to underwrite the trial. A nonprofit organization will underwrite the trial only if the disease is common enough to justify spending the limited and valuable resources needed to perform the trial. And particularly with treatments that are widely used, relatively innocuous, and not regulated (such as many of the Eastern herbal therapies), the companies that make the products may not wish to have a product study take place, for fear that the study may prove that the product does *not* work. They may not want to find out.

The decision to participate in a clinical trial should be individualized, based on the overall risk-to-benefit ratio for an individual patient, and interpreted within the context of other, more standard, treatment options that may have a more predictable (although not necessarily higher) likelihood of benefit and known side effects. That being said, by participating in clinical trials, patients can contribute in an important way to the advancement of medical science and potentially receive an effective treatment for their disease in the process.

A Personal Perspective on Managing Chemotherapy Side Effects

Angel S. Gnau

When I was diagnosed with ovarian cancer in March 2006, I had carboplatin/pacli-taxel combination chemotherapy after debulking surgery. This is still the standard chemotherapy given in first-line treatment today.

I had an almost five-year remission. However, the cancer recurred in 2011, 2013, and 2014. Along with the carbo/Taxol [carboplatin/paclitaxel], I have had cis-platin, gemcitabine, doxorubicin, the oral drug tamoxifen, and weekly Taxol.

Here are the side effects I encountered and how I managed them:

Changes in taste—Many patients report having a metal taste in their mouth. For me, everything tasted like cardboard, which made eating well that much harder. I found using spices and condiments such as mustard, ketchup, and bar-becue sauces really helped bring out taste. It is best to use a mild toothpaste and mouthwash such as Biotene.

Constipation—After a little trial and error, I learned what I needed to do for the constipation. For me, it ended up being a combination of two to three stool softeners a day, prune juice, MiraLax, and sometimes a mild laxative such as senna.

Fatigue—This is a common issue with most of the chemotherapy drugs. As the drugs kill the cancer cells, they kill many healthy, fast-growing cells as well. Get lots of rest. Don't push yourself. Your body will let you know when to rest. Listen to it.

Hair loss—Not all drugs cause hair loss. When hair starts falling out, usually about one to three weeks after beginning treatment, have your hair cut short so it is easier to deal with and not as noticeable as it continues to fall. Once it starts coming out in clumps, it is usually best to shave it. Plan ahead and buy some head coverings or a wig *before* you lose all your hair. Make sure to have sleeping caps. Bald heads get cold! I also use a neck warmer in the winter.

Low white blood cell and platelet counts—Low counts are common with many drugs. While I tried eating mushrooms, taking shark oil, and other home remedies to boost platelets, nothing really worked. For low white count, the doctor can prescribe Neulasta or Neupogen to boost count.

Nausea—This is less of an issue today with antiemetic medicines such as ondansetron (Zofran), prochlorperazine (Compazine), promethazine (Phenergan), and others. Don't wait until you get sick to take something; get in front of it and take antinausea medicine at the slightest hint of nausea. If you know you are prone to nausea, take it *before* nausea sets in.

Neuropathy—This was mild for me on Taxol, but some women are severely affected by it. There are drugs that are useful for the treatment of neuropathy, but I never needed them. I did take L-glutamine for a bit, mainly to build muscle, but I understand it can be used for neuropathy.

Rash—With Doxil or doxorubicin, rash is common. Icing hands and feet during chemo may help. The rash started out slow and built up for me until it was covering almost my entire body. Stay out of the sun and don't use hot water. Friction can cause rash as well. My dermatologist prescribed triamcinolone 0.1% for the rash, and it helped tremendously.

CHAPTER 4

The Side Effects of Chemotherapy

Sharon D. Thompson, BSN, OCN

<hr>

You don't choose how you're going to die, or when.
You can only decide how you're going to live. Now.

—Joan Baez

In the previous two chapters we described surgery and chemotherapy as treatments for women with ovarian cancer. Our goal when we treat women with ovarian cancer is to remove all the disease with surgery, if possible, and treat any microscopic or remaining disease with chemotherapy. The goal of chemotherapy for newly diagnosed patients is cure, with remission and increased survival time as alternative goals.

When we consider chemotherapy regimens for our patients, the woman's quality of life is just as important as the effectiveness of the treatment. If you're being treated for ovarian cancer, you should discuss with your doctor and nurse any side effects that you experience, even if the side effect seems to be just a nuisance. Health care providers need to know about all their patients' side effects in order to prevent or decrease complications that can interfere with day-to-day living or long-term health.

Many side effects from chemotherapy occur because the chemotherapy attacks both the rapidly dividing cancer cells and normal cells (as discussed in chapter 3). Most side effects (for example, low blood counts) are temporary, lasting only days or weeks after the chemotherapy treatment, while others (such as hair loss) resolve after the chemotherapy treatments have been completed. On rare occasions, however, the side effects may be long term or permanent. Hearing loss and *peripheral neuropathy* (numbness in the fingers and hands or the toes and feet) are two examples of permanent side effects.

Every person reacts individually to chemotherapy, and side effects may be difficult to predict. Also, different chemotherapy agents cause different side effects. Symptoms of side effects can be mild and may not interfere with daily life. If side effects become severe, chemotherapy treatment may be interrupted or delayed, and the woman may need to be admitted to the hospital. Short delays do not necessarily interfere with the overall effects of treatment. Since each person responds differently to chemotherapy, your doctor and nurse will decide the best recommendation for your situation.

If side effects are recognized early, it is easier to decrease their severity, prevent them in the future, and avoid the risk of potential life-threatening complications. In this chapter, we discuss the most common side effects of chemotherapy as well as how to manage them.

Low White Blood Cell Counts (Leukopenia)

As noted in chapter 3, a complete blood count (CBC) will be done before each course of chemotherapy to monitor the patient's response to the treatment. One of the most dangerous side effects from chemotherapy is low white blood cell (WBC) counts, a condition called *leukopenia*. White blood cells help fight infection, and a patient with low WBC counts is at greater risk of infection than normal. A low neutrophil count (*neutropenia*) is of special concern, because neutrophils are the biggest infection-fighting WBCs. Many of the agents used in treating ovarian cancer cause white blood cell levels to decline (see table 4.1). The risk of infection is generally greatest seven to fourteen days after chemotherapy is administered; however, the risk may continue up to three or four weeks after treatment.

TABLE 4.1 *Chemotherapy Used in Ovarian Cancer That Increases the Risk for Low White Blood Cell Count*

Capecitabine (Xeloda)	Gemcitabine (Gemzar)
Carboplatin	Ifosfamide (Ifex)
Cisplatin	Liposomal doxorubicin (Doxil)
Cyclophosphamide (Cytoxan)	Oxaliplatin (Eloxatin)
Docetaxel (Taxotere)	Paclitaxel (Taxol)
Doxorubicin (Adriamycin)	Topotecan (Hycamtin)
Etoposide (VP-16)	Vinorelbine (Navelbine)

Low white blood cell counts do not necessarily mean you have an infection or will get one. If you are receiving chemotherapy, however, you need to be aware of the common symptoms of infection, including fever and chills (see table 4.2). Your doctor and nurse will watch your condition carefully for any sign of infection, but you are your own closest monitor, and you should contact your health care provider if you have any symptoms. (*Symptoms* are what you as the patient experience; *signs* are what the doctor finds on examination.)

A decrease in the WBC count is a temporary side effect of chemotherapy, generally lasting up to ten days and returning to normal in three to four weeks at most. Some doctors obtain a complete blood count to check when the *nadir* (lowest level) of the WBC count occurs, approximately seven to fourteen days after chemotherapy. This information may be important in providing you with preventive instructions or medications to reduce the risk of infection. The doctor may also prescribe an antibiotic to prevent infection or to treat an existing infection.

White blood cell counts are rechecked before each scheduled chemotherapy treatment. If WBCs are low, chemotherapy may be postponed until the counts return to a safe level. If treatment is postponed due to low WBC counts, the provider may prescribe a medication, called *myeloid growth factor*, to help increase the WBC and neutrophil counts. There are several formulations of this medication available, and it is given by injection just under the skin; its purpose is to assist the patient's bone marrow in increasing production of WBCs. Myeloid growth factor may also be given preventively to patients whose prescribed chemotherapy regimen is known to cause severe neutro-

TABLE 4.2   *Common Symptoms of Infection*

Fever higher than 100.5°F
Redness, drainage, tenderness, or swelling (especially from wound or
   catheter site)
Sore throat with white patches on throat or tongue
Burning with urination; bloody or cloudy urine
Productive cough
Chills
Ear pain
Headache or severe sinus pain
Stiff or sore neck
Skin rash

penia. Your provider or nurse will inform you of the scheduling of this injection and the potential side effects.

Patient Education for Infection Risk

- Wash your hands with soap and warm water. Always wash your hands after using the restroom, before cooking and eating, when taking care of pets, and after you have been in a public place. Use hand sanitizer only when soap and water are not available.
- Have everyone around you wash their hands with soap and warm water.
- Bathe daily and keep yourself clean. If you have a catheter, keep the area around it clean and dry.
- Brush your teeth after meals and before going to bed.
- Avoid large crowds and crowded rooms where infection may be spread. This is especially important between seven and fourteen days after each chemotherapy treatment, when you are at greatest risk of infection.
- Wash raw fruits and vegetables before cooking or eating. Cook meats and eggs completely, to avoid consuming bacteria due to undercooking.
- Avoid people who have infections (colds, flu, chicken pox, and so on).

- Avoid people who may have just received a live vaccine (such as chicken pox, polio, or measles vaccine).
- Avoid cuts or breaks in the skin. If you have a cut, wash the area immediately and monitor it for signs of infection (redness, discharge, swelling, and so on).
- Minimize the use of any medications that may mask a fever, such as aspirin, acetaminophen, or ibuprofen.
- If you are in a sexual relationship, talk with your doctor or nurse about any precautions you should take. If your WBC counts are very low, you may be asked to refrain from oral sex or penile intercourse for a short time. Using a condom may be recommended to help prevent infection.

When to Call Your Doctor or Nurse

- If you have a temperature of 100.5°F or greater. If you have chills, please take your temperature.
- If you have any other symptoms of infection, such as cough; sore throat; ear pain; headache or severe sinus pain; stiff neck; skin rash; sores or white coating on your tongue or mouth; burning or pain with urination; cloudy or bloody urine; or redness, swelling, or drainage from a wound or catheter site.

Low Red Blood Cell Counts (Anemia)

A person with anemia is not producing enough red blood cells (RBCs). Women who have had surgery and are receiving chemotherapy or radiation therapy (see chapter 5) for ovarian cancer are at risk of developing anemia. We monitor our patients closely for anemia and other side effects of chemotherapy.

When anemia develops gradually over a long time, women may be unaware that they have the condition, although some women experience fatigue and weakness as the primary symptom of anemia. Oxygen is carried in red blood cells, and when the number of cells is reduced, low oxygen levels in the bloodstream can cause fatigue. Information on levels of RBCs, hemoglobin (Hgb), and hematocrit (Hct) is provided by the complete blood count. (Hemoglobin and hematocrit are laboratory results that reflect essentially the same thing—the level of RBCs.)

There are many other symptoms besides fatigue and weakness that women with anemia may experience (see table 4.3). Other symptoms of anemia include headache, dizziness, shortness of breath— especially during physical activity—or a rapid heartbeat. If you are being treated for ovarian cancer and experience any symptoms of anemia, you should report these symptoms to your doctor or nurse.

Unlike with neutropenia, it is not necessary to delay or postpone chemotherapy if a woman becomes anemic, although she may feel too tired or just not feel well enough to receive treatment. For patients experiencing severe or prolonged anemia, the physician may order additional testing to determine the cause of the anemia. Besides chemotherapy, bleeding, low iron, kidney dysfunction, or inherited conditions may be the cause of the anemia. If chemotherapy is identified as the cause, additional treatment for the anemia may be recommended, to improve the patient's symptoms. *Erythropoiesis-stimulating agents* (ESAs) and red blood cell transfusions are two treatments that may be prescribed. ESAs are injections given to patients weekly or monthly to stimulate the body to produce more RBCs. ESAs typically improve RBC counts very gradually over many weeks and therefore may not decrease fatigue quickly. RBC transfusions can rapidly increase the number of RBCs and therefore improve fatigue quickly. Both of these treatments for anemia have risks and benefits. Your provider will determine which option is best to treat your anemia, based on your individual circumstances. The risk of acquiring the human immunodeficiency virus (HIV) after blood transfusion is estimated to be 1 in 1.5 million, according to the Centers for Disease

TABLE 4.3 *Symptoms of Anemia*

Fatigue	Irritability
Dizziness	Decreased ability to concentrate
Headache	Indigestion
Shortness of breath with activity	Lack of appetite
Feeling cold	Paleness of skin
Fast heartbeat	Weakness

Control and Prevention. Thus, a blood transfusion is generally safe, but the decision to administer a transfusion is not made lightly.

Patient Education for Anemia

- Report any symptoms of anemia to your doctor or nurse.
- Conserve your energy. Choose the most important things to complete in your day. Typically, it is best to perform the most difficult tasks early in the day, when you have the most energy.
- Allow friends and family members to help when they offer.
- Prevent injury. If you are anemic, you may not heal as well or as quickly as you normally would.
- If you are dizzy, change position slowly from sitting to standing. Do not drive if you feel dizzy.
- Balance rest with activity. Take short naps during the day. Be careful not to sleep too much during the day as this may make sleep difficult at night.
- Take short walks and exercise a little every day.
- Maintain proper nutrition. Discuss with your doctor or nurse if you should increase high-protein or high-iron foods in your diet to improve cell repair.
- Drink more water and other fluids daily.
- Discuss the need for ESAs or blood transfusions with your doctor.

Low Platelet Counts and Bleeding (Thrombocytopenia)

Platelets are produced in your bone marrow and are a component of your blood responsible for clotting. If you have a decreased platelet count (called *thrombocytopenia*), you are at increased risk for bleeding in the form of easy bruising after minor trauma or excessive blood loss from a minor cut. Chemotherapy and radiation are common causes of low platelets. The platelet count generally decreases between one to three weeks after administration of chemotherapy and may take two to six weeks to return to normal levels. The normal platelet count is approximately 150,000 to 400,000/mm^3. If your platelet levels remain low at the time chemotherapy is scheduled, treatment may be delayed or the dose modified. It is important to know that platelets may be transfused in a person who has severely low platelets. Your doctor will discuss this possibility if needed.

Patient Education for Bleeding

- Report any excessive bleeding or bruises to your doctor or nurse. In addition, report skin changes such as tiny red pinpoint spots on your skin, bad headaches, vision changes, or mental confusion.
- If you are informed by your provider that your platelets are low, you should protect yourself from any activities that may increase your risk for injury or bleeding. Use electric shavers, avoid sharp objects such as scissors or knives, wear shoes at all times, avoid sports (such as roller skating or bike riding), and brush with a soft bristle toothbrush. Avoid tooth flossing, picking scabs, and inserting things in your rectum or vagina (not even thermometers, enema tips, or tampons), and blow your nose gently.
- Avoid elective procedures that may increase the risk for bleeding, such as dental cleaning and other dental procedures, placement of a PICC line or central catheter, a biopsy, or acupuncture. (A PICC is a *peripherally inserted central catheter*. It is similar to a central catheter but the tubing extends from the arm instead of under the collarbone.)
- Prevent constipation and avoid bearing down with bowel movements. Use stool softeners and laxatives as needed. Report any rectal bleeding to your provider immediately.
- Talk with your doctor or nurse before you take any new medications, herbal supplements, or vitamins. Avoid medications that increase your risk of bleeding, such as aspirin, ibuprofen, digoxin, furosemide, heparin, and warfarin.
- If there are repeated delays in your chemotherapy, your doctor may prescribe a reduced dosage of your treatment to prevent future treatment delays or dangerous side effects.
- If you begin bleeding, apply pressure on the area with a clean

cloth until the bleeding stops. If you bruise after trauma, apply ice on the area of injury for about 20 minutes.

Nausea and Vomiting

Chemotherapy-induced nausea and vomiting (CINV) may be mild, moderate, or severe. Chemotherapy drugs are classified according to each drug's known potential for causing nausea and vomiting. Similarly, the drugs your provider chooses to treat CINV will be based on the dosage and kind of chemotherapy you are receiving. Not all chemotherapy agents cause nausea (see table 4.4). The feeling of being queasy and unable to eat or drink can be unpleasant and can lead to physical problems like poor nutrition and poor hydration. The goal is to prevent CINV before it occurs.

The risks posed by prolonged CINV are dehydration and kidney problems. CINV may also decrease a woman's energy level, interfere with her ability to perform daily activities, and adversely affect her quality of life. If nausea or vomiting is not controlled, and dehydration or other potential problems exist, the patient may receive intravenous fluids in the doctor's office or the treatment center.

CINV can be further classified into the following types: anticipatory nausea, acute nausea and vomiting, and delayed nausea. Different classes of drugs are used to treat each of the three different kinds of chemotherapy-induced nausea and vomiting (see table 4.5). If you do not get relief from your antinausea medication, notify your doctor or nurse sooner rather than later, so another drug can be prescribed.

TABLE 4.4 *Chemotherapy Used in Ovarian Cancer That Increases the Risk for Nausea and Vomiting*

Cisplatin (can also cause delayed nausea up to 4 days)
Cyclophosphamide (Cytoxan) (delayed nausea can last several days)
Altretamine (Hexalen)
Ifosfamide (Ifex)
Oxaliplatin (Eloxatin)
Administration of a combination of chemotherapy agents

TABLE 4.5 *Medications for Chemotherapy-Induced Nausea and Vomiting*

Class, Generic, and Brand Names	Common Side Effects	Uses
Benzodiazepines Diazepam (Valium) Lorazepam (Ativan)	Sedation, confusion, amnesia	Anticipatory CINV, anxiety
Phenothiazines Prochlorperazine (Compazine) Promethazine (Phenergan) Trimethobenzamide (Tigan)	Sedation, confusion, involuntary muscle movements (can be prevented with diphenhydramine)	Acute and delayed CINV
Benzamides Metoclopramide (Reglan)	Sedation, diarrhea, anxiety, involuntary muscle movements (can be prevented with diphenhydramine)	Acute and delayed CINV
5-HT$_3$ antagonists Dolasetron (Anzemet) Granisetron (Kytril) Ondansetron (Zofran) Palonosetron (Aloxi)	Headache, constipation, blurry vision with ondansetron	Acute CINV
Steroids Dexamethasone (Decadron)	Euphoria, insomnia, edema, facial flushing if given in IV quickly; may cause perineal burning	Acute and delayed CINV
Antihistamines Diphenhydramine (Benadryl)	Sedation, dry mouth, dizziness; some patients have reported restlessness	Delayed CINV
Butyrophenones Haloperidol (Haldol) Droperidol (Inapsine)	Sedation, low blood pressure, involuntary muscle movements	Delayed CINV
Cannabinoids Dronabinol (Marinol, THC)	Sedation, dizziness, euphoria, paranoia, dry mouth, visual changes	Delayed CINV
Anticholinergics Scopolamine patch (Scopoderm)	Sedation, dry mouth, restlessness, headache	Anticipatory and delayed CINV

continued

TABLE 4.5   *continued*

Class, Generic, and Brand Names	Common Side Effects	Uses
Neurokinin-1 receptor antagonists Aprepitant (oral Emend) Fosaprepitant (IV Emend)	Fatigue, constipation, diarrhea, hiccups	In combination with other antiemetics for acute and delayed CINV

Anticipatory Nausea

Anticipatory nausea occurs when the patient feels sick or throws up *before* receiving chemotherapy. This is a learned response and is associated with remembering a previous incident of being sick after a chemotherapy treatment. Some patients say they feel sick to their stomach if they simply drive by the treatment center.

To avoid anticipatory nausea and vomiting, your provider may recommend taking an antianxiety medication such as lorazepam 30 to 60 minutes before chemotherapy. As noted in chapter 3, for patients who have had a particularly difficult time with nausea during previous chemotherapy cycles, it is often recommended to start the antinausea medication the night before treatment and continue it the morning of the infusion.

Acute CINV

This type of nausea and vomiting occurs within the first 18 to 24 hours of receiving a chemotherapy treatment. The medications recommended for avoiding or alleviating acute chemotherapy-induced nausea and vomiting are a class of drugs, called 5-HT$_3$ *antagonists,* that work to block the receptors in the brain that cause CINV. This class of drugs is most effective when taken the day of chemotherapy and up to two or three days after chemotherapy.

Four different 5-HT$_3$ antagonists are used to treat acute CINV: dolasetron, granisetron, ondansetron, and palonosetron. They are recommended for women receiving chemotherapy drugs that cause moderate to severe CINV. They can be given orally or intravenously at the same time chemotherapy is administered. They do not cause drowsiness but may have other side effects, such as constipation or headache. Your doctor or nurse will discuss the side effects of the medications with you. Depending on the CINV potential of your specific chemotherapy regimen, your doctor may also prescribe additional drugs such as steroids or neurokinin-1 receptor antagonists to help control chemotherapy-induced nausea and vomiting.

Delayed Nausea

Delayed nausea and vomiting occurs 18 to 24 hours after chemotherapy treatment and can last up to four days. Cisplatin produces nausea more than the other chemotherapy agents, and the nausea is often delayed. Carboplatin may be substituted because women experience less chemotherapy-induced nausea and vomiting with this drug. However, carboplatin has the disadvantage of causing more severe decreases in the blood counts (WBC and platelets). Decisions about which cytotoxic agents to use are made for each individual, depending on how she tolerates the chemotherapy.

Delayed nausea is a challenging side effect because the patient may stop taking the prescribed antinausea medications if she has no immediate nausea or vomiting, only to experience nausea three days later. Thus, if you are prescribed a medication for delayed nausea, we recommend that you take it even if you are not vomiting or feeling nauseated.

There are many choices for treating delayed CINV. For chemotherapy that causes moderate to severe CINV, prochlorperazine or metoclopramide are recommended in combination with a low-dose steroid such as dexamethasone. No single standard treatment is recognized for delayed CINV, and providers take different approaches to overcoming this side effect of chemotherapy. There are many options, so if one medication does not control delayed nausea and vomiting, another one can be started. Instead of switching to new medications for delayed CINV, some patients continue to take the medications they took in the acute setting—and that's fine, as long as the symptoms are relieved. Drugs such as prochlorperazine, lorazepam or metoclopramide may cause drowsiness, and the 5-HT$_3$ drugs are significantly more expensive. Your provider will decide on an individual basis which drugs are best to treat your delayed chemotherapy-induced nausea and vomiting.

Patient Education for Nausea and Vomiting

- Take the prescribed antinausea medications exactly as directed by your doctor and nurse. If you do not understand the schedule for taking the medications, or if you do not understand other aspects of how to take the medications, talk to your doctor or nurse.
- Contact your doctor or nurse
  - if you are unable to eat or drink fluids due to uncontrolled nausea and vomiting,
  - if nausea and vomiting keep you from doing things you want to do, or
  - if you lose more than two pounds in one day.
- Inform your doctor or nurse if your urine is dark, or if you are not urinating as often as you normally do. (Dark urine and infrequent urination are signs of dehydration.)
- Eating and drinking are best done 30 to 60 minutes after taking antinausea medication. Eat less greasy, fried, salty, sweet, or spicy food. Choose bland foods such as soups, chicken, cereal, crackers, oatmeal, pasta, potatoes, rice, toast, bananas, gelatin, yogurt, popsicles, and canned fruits, as they are easier to digest.
- Eat five or six small meals during the day, instead of three larger meals.
- Reduce odors (hot foods, perfumes, chemicals) that can cause nausea.
- If possible, have someone else cook your meals for you. If this is not possible, freeze several meals before chemotherapy so that you can reheat them when you do not feel up to cooking.
- Take small sips of water during the day if you find it hard to drink a full glass at one time. It is most important to increase fluid intake, especially during the first three to five days following chemotherapy treatment, so you do not get dehydrated.

- Relaxation techniques, meditation, deep breathing, visualization tapes, music therapy, and acupuncture or acupressure are nondrug approaches that have been shown to help control CINV. Discuss these alternative options with your nurse or social worker, who can provide instruction, videotapes, or audiotapes for you and can point you in the right direction for more resources.

Constipation

There are many causes of constipation, and many women have irregular or hard bowel movements, or difficulty moving their bowels, even without a cancer diagnosis. When a woman is being treated for ovarian cancer, however, she is likely to develop constipation, for any of the following reasons:

1 decreased dietary fiber and fluids due to side effects from chemotherapy, such as nausea or vomiting
2 reduced activity levels due to effects of surgery or fatigue
3 compression of the lumen (opening) of the bowel due to tumor or scar tissue (adhesions)
4 administration of chemotherapy agents known to cause constipation (see table 4.6)
5 administration of pain medications, antidepressants, diuretics, iron and calcium supplements, or the antinausea medication 5-HT$_3$ antagonists, which often cause constipation

If there is any suspicion that a bowel obstruction is the cause of the constipation, contact your doctor or nurse immediately. Symptoms of a bowel obstruction include nausea and vomiting (especially after eating), inability to pass gas, increasing abdominal girth and discomfort, and constipation.

TABLE 4.6 *Chemotherapy Used in Ovarian Cancer That Increases the Risk for Constipation*

Altretamine (Hexalen)	Cisplatin
Topotecan (Hycamtin)	Paclitaxel (Taxol)
Vinorelbine (Vinorelbine)	

A regular bowel routine, including appropriate dietary habits and hydration, adequate activity level, and incorporating medications, all play a role in bowel regularity. The goal is to maintain a regular schedule for bowel elimination, and if possible, to prevent constipation from starting. Constipation can be prevented by eating high-fiber foods such as whole-grain breads and cereals, fruits and vegetables, and nuts and seeds. In addition, drinking at least eight glasses of liquid every day ensures enough fluids to prevent dehydration. Walking or riding an exercise bike for 15 to 30 minutes daily is a great way to maintain the normal movement of the intestines.

If you become constipated, your doctor or nurse may recommend that you try one of the many preparations available to address this problem (see table 4.7). These include bulk producers, saline laxatives, osmotic laxatives, detergent laxatives, and stimulant-type laxatives. Many people without illness manage constipation using their own judgment with over-the-counter products. Among the many products available, most people find one that comfortably relieves occasional constipation. Table 4.8 describes one regimen recommended for treating constipation.

Bulk products, such as psyllium (Metamucil), should be taken with large amounts of water. If you are not able to drink large volumes of water or fluid, the bulk products are not the best choice for you. In addition, although bulk products are effective at *keeping* individuals regular, once constipation has developed, especially if there has been no bowel movement for several days, a bulk product may add to the

TABLE 4.7 *Laxatives for Chemotherapy-Induced Constipation*

Bisacodyl (Correctol, Dulcolax)
Docusate sodium (Colace)
Lactulose (Chronulac, Cephulac)
Magnesium citrate (Milk of Magnesia)
Methylcellulose (Citrucel)
Polycarbophil (FiberCon)
Polyethylene glycol (MiraLax)
Psyllium (Fiberall, Metamucil)
Senna (Senokot, Ex-Lax)
Sodium phosphate (Fleet enema, Fleet Phospho-Soda)

NOTE: Table 4.8 lists specific "dos and don'ts" for using these preparations.

TABLE 4.8   *Common Regimens to Treat Constipation*

Do not take any medication unless approved by your doctor.

Take 2 Senna-S pills at bedtime.

If more than 2 bowel movements occur the next day:
Reduce dose to 1 pill at bedtime.

If no bowel movement:
Increase Senna-S to 4 pills at bedtime (or 2 pills in morning, 2 pills at night).

If bowel movement occurs:
Continue same routine.

If no bowel movement:
Increase Senna-S to 6 to 8 pills at bedtime.

If still no bowel movement:
Call doctor or nurse and make sure there is no impaction.

If no impaction, add one of the following:
Bisacodyl tablet (may cause cramping)
Lactulose or polyethylene glycol
Magnesium citrate

---

problem by bulking up the stool and making it more difficult to pass. (Bulk products are effective for individuals with loose stool, to help give it form.)

Stool softeners are used to soften the stool as it passes through the bowel. A softener alone may not effectively stimulate a bowel movement, so both a laxative and a softener should be used.

Stimulant-type laxatives, such as bisacodyl (Dulcolax), may be prescribed and are generally effective, although they may cause cramping. These agents are the most commonly prescribed medications for treating narcotic-induced constipation.

Osmotic laxatives, such as polyethylene glycol (MiraLax), are made of synthetic sugar molecules. They stimulate a bowel movement by drawing fluid into the bowel as they pass into the colon undigested.

Enemas can be helpful for removing stool from the lower colon, but if constipation has been chronic or there has been no bowel movement for several days, it may be better to take an oral product, which can stimulate the entire bowel. Enemas should not be used by anyone with a low white blood cell count or low platelet count due to the risk of infection and rectal bleeding.

Patient Education for Constipation

- Talk with your doctor or nurse about your regular bowel pattern and how likely it is that your chemotherapy regimen will cause constipation.
- Increase your fluid intake to eight 8-ounce glasses a day, if possible.
- Eat foods high in fiber and bulk (bran, whole grains, legumes, fruits and vegetables).
- Increase activity by walking (around the neighborhood, around the mall, and so on), joining a gym, or obtaining a referral to physical therapy for an exercise training program.
- Follow your doctor or nurse's recommendation for bowel routine. You may need to take a laxative or a stool softener (or both) daily, and you may need to increase the amount you take as time goes on.
- If you are taking pain medications, you may need to increase the dose of laxatives with each increase in pain medication.
- Try to move your bowels at the same time every day (for example, after breakfast).
- Call your doctor or nurse if you have not had a bowel movement in two days, or if you have nausea and vomiting, inability to pass gas, abdominal pain, or abdominal *distension* (bloating).

Diarrhea

Diarrhea is defined as more than two loose bowel movements daily. It is not a common side effect for women with ovarian cancer or for women who are being treated for ovarian cancer, but diarrhea may become a problem for someone who has had surgery on the bowel, has received pelvic radiation, or is getting certain types of chemotherapy. The chemotherapy agents used in treating ovarian cancer that most commonly cause diarrhea are fluorouracil, irinotecan, and capecitabine (see table 4.9).

Diarrhea can be a sign of a *fecal impaction*. A fecal impaction occurs when hard stool is unable to pass normally through the rectum, and loose stool seeps around the stool mass, with "diarrhea" the result. In this situation, laxatives and stool softeners are the treatment of choice. A rectal examination can confirm a fecal impaction.

Other causes of diarrhea are lactose (dairy product) intolerance and other food intolerance. Lactose intolerance can be an inherited condition, or it can develop as a result of repeated infections or chemotherapy. Removing dairy products from your diet or using lactase enzymes or drops may stop the diarrhea.

Inflammatory bowel disease, anxiety, antibiotic use, and use of antacids containing magnesium can also cause diarrhea. Diarrhea is sometimes an indication of a viral or a bacterial infection, especially if antidiarrheal medications do not control the stool output. Signs of infection include fever, watery bowel movements, or stool that contains mucus or blood. A stool culture can identify an infection.

Patient Education for Diarrhea

- Inform your doctor or nurse if you have more than two loose stools a day for more than 24 hours.
- Inform your doctor or nurse if you have a fever higher than 100.5°F, if your stool is watery or bloody, or if it contains mucus.
- Inform your doctor or nurse if, in addition to diarrhea, you have decreased urine output, dizziness, weakness, or muscle

TABLE 4.9 *Chemotherapy Used in Ovarian Cancer That Increases the Risk for Diarrhea*

Fluorouracil (5-FU)
Capecitabine (Xeloda)
Liposomal doxorubicin (Doxil)
Irinotecan (Camptosar)
Other targeted therapy agents

cramps, which may be a sign of dehydration or loss of electrolytes.

- Discuss other causes of the diarrhea with your doctor or nurse.
- Begin an over-the-counter antidiarrheal product, such as loperamide (Imodium), as directed by your provider. If your diarrhea does not decrease or clear up with over-the-counter products, your doctor may write a prescription for a stronger antidiarrheal, such as diphenoxylate and atropine (Lomotil).
- If your diarrhea continues for more than three or four days while taking antidiarrheal medication, a stool culture should be performed to check for infection.
- If you have diarrhea, avoid high-fiber foods, caffeine, alcoholic drinks, spicy and greasy foods, citrus drinks, dairy products, gas-forming foods, and fruit, as these foods can make diarrhea worse.
- Maintain a low-residue diet until the diarrhea clears up. (A *low-residue diet* consists of low-fiber foods that are easy for your body to digest and that reduce the amount of stool in the colon.) The BRAT diet (a specific low-residue diet) is commonly recommended when someone has diarrhea (bananas, rice, applesauce, and toast).
- Hydrate yourself with sports drinks that contain electrolytes. Other choices include Pedialyte, rice soups, Jell-O, and broth.
- Keep the skin around the rectum clean and dry to avoid irritation. Vaseline and skin barrier creams, both available without a prescription, may offer soothing relief.

Hair Loss (Alopecia)

Alopecia is a general term for any loss of hair (the Greek word *alōpekia* means "loss of hair"). *Alopecia totalis* is the term used when a person loses all of his or her scalp hair, while *alopecia universalis* refers to losing all hair from the body. Chemotherapy may cause loss of scalp and body hair, depending on the specific drug. Hair loss as a side effect of chemotherapy occurs because chemotherapy drugs attack rapidly dividing cells, including hair follicles.

Not all chemotherapy causes total hair loss. Some chemotherapy agents cause only thinning of the hair, and some agents do not cause any hair loss at all (see table 4.10). Approximately 15 to 20 percent of people undergoing chemotherapy will lose eyelashes, eyebrows, and underarm and pubic hair in addition to the hair from the head. Some patients report a sore or tingling scalp before or during hair shedding.

Generally, hair loss begins about two to three weeks after the start of chemotherapy. The hair begins to thin and fall out in uneven patches or strands, as noticed on the pillow and when washing hair. There are no known treatments (such as ice caps or lotions) that are effective in preventing alopecia if the chemotherapy agent is known to cause hair loss. Infrequent washing and brushing of hair will keep hair from falling out faster but will not prevent it from falling out altogether. Hair regrowth usually begins four to eight weeks after the drug is discontinued. Sometimes the new hair growth can be curlier, straighter, or even a different color than your hair before chemotherapy.

The emotional toll of alopecia is often underestimated. Hair loss can have a profound psychological impact on an individual—so profound that she refuses treatment. Even though the hair will return, the loss of hair is a constant reminder of cancer to many patients. Women with long hair are advised to cut it short before beginning chemotherapy, to decrease the psychological effect of loss. Cutting their hair or shaving their head with an electric razor is seen by some patients as a way to maintain some control during treatment.

Many hospitals and cancer centers offer support groups and classes on beauty and body image. The American Cancer Society provides a free national public service program called "Look Good Feel Better," which teaches women beauty techniques to improve their appearance and self-image during chemotherapy. It may also be help-

TABLE 4.10 *Chemotherapy Used in Ovarian Cancer That Increases the Risk for Hair Loss*

Cyclophosphamide (Cytoxan)	Paclitaxel (Taxol)
Topotecan (Hycamtin)*	Docetaxel (Taxotere)
Ifosfamide (Ifex)	Etoposide (VP-16)
Doxorubicin (Adriamycin)	

*Hair loss varies.

ful for emotional support to join a support group to talk with other patients who have alopecia. Shopping for wigs, scarves, or hats before the hair loss is recommended. Wigs are paid for by many health insurance policies. Discuss this possibility with your doctor, nurse, or social worker and be sure to obtain a prescription for a "cranial prosthesis."

Sun sensitivity is a concern for women with alopecia. Be sure to protect your head and eyes from the sun by using sunscreen and wearing a hat and sunglasses. In the colder months, it is just as important to cover your head to prevent loss of body heat, even while indoors, for your comfort.

Patient Education for Alopecia

- Discuss with your doctor or nurse if the prescribed chemotherapy will cause alopecia.
- Select wigs, hats, and scarves before hair loss begins to occur. Choosing a wig or hairpiece while you still have hair can help match the color to your hair.
- Wash your hair gently with a mild shampoo and pat it dry with a soft towel.
- Consider cutting your hair short or shaving your scalp prior to hair loss. If you decide to shave your head, be sure to use an electric razor so you won't cut your scalp.
- Protect your head, eyes, and face from the sun with sunscreen, head coverings, and sunglasses.
- Ask your doctor for a prescription for a wig, because a prescription is needed for insurance purposes. The prescription should read: "Cranial prosthesis for chemotherapy-induced alopecia." Not all insurance companies will cover this expense.

Fatigue

Fatigue (lack of energy, feeling tired, wanting to sleep a lot) is one of the most common side effects of cancer and cancer treatment. Fatigue may also be a symptom of the cancer. It may even be the symptom that brought the patient to visit a doctor in the first place, before cancer was diagnosed. Surgery causes fatigue, and recovery can take weeks to months in many cases. When chemotherapy or radiation is added after the surgery, fatigue may become overwhelming, especially in the first month or two, and may even worsen as treatment continues. Radiation-caused fatigue may be noticed by patients as early as the third week of radiation treatment. Fatigue may last up to six months after radiation is completed. During chemotherapy, fatigue may worsen throughout treatment and can be constant until treatment is completed. For some patients, fatigue may last up to a year after completion of chemotherapy.

There are many other causes of fatigue in addition to the direct effects of illness and treatment. Lifestyle can play a role in fatigue, as can a large dose of daily responsibilities (such as employment, housework, caring for family, and financial concerns). People who do not get enough sleep, as well as people who get too much sleep, often report not having any energy. Poor dietary habits and lack of adequate nutrition and hydration can easily cause a person to feel tired and weak. Too much exercise, and not enough rest for the muscles between workouts, can cause fatigue, and so can a lack of exercise and activity. For most people, increasing activity (within reason) is an excellent way to increase energy levels.

If you are recovering from cancer and cancer treatment, we encourage you to maintain your daily routine as closely as possible. Keeping up your daily routine can reduce chronic feelings of fatigue. Even if you need to rest after showering and dressing and are moving more slowly than usual, activity will keep your circulation healthy and prevent your muscles from weakening. Some patients keep a journal so they can identify their energy patterns and plan their activities or social events around their fatigue.

Fatigue is difficult to measure and may not be thought of as an important symptom. One way to measure your fatigue is to gauge how it interferes with your life. Tell your doctor or nurse how fatigue is affecting your life. Use a numerical scale from 0 to 10 to describe your fatigue as it affects you daily, with 0 being no fatigue, and 10 being the worst fatigue you can imagine or have ever experienced. Discuss how your feelings of fatigue affect your mood, your daily activities, your concentration, and your ability to work or care for yourself and your family. Your doctor and nurse will want to know if the fatigue came on suddenly, which may indicate a serious problem, or gradually, which is common with treatment-related fatigue. Medical causes of fatigue include anemia and electrolyte imbalances, which can be caused by dehydration, vomiting, and diarrhea. These two conditions can be identified through a routine blood test and can be treated. Depression and pain can also cause symptoms of fatigue.

Patient Education for Fatigue

- Tell your doctor and nurse how fatigue is interfering with your lifestyle and activities of daily living.
- Rate your fatigue on a scale of 0 to 10, with 0 meaning no fatigue, and 10 meaning severe fatigue.
- Keep a journal of your fatigue as it relates to treatment and activity.
- Report any factors that appear to be related to your fatigue, such as headache, feeling cold, feeling dizzy, or becoming short of breath with activity. These are symptoms of anemia.
- Discuss the cause of your fatigue with your doctor or nurse. Unless there is a reason for you not to increase your activity level, doing so may help to decrease feelings of fatigue. Walk around the house or walk around the block. Once you can walk this far, increase walking time by 10 minutes each week. Stretching, yoga, or Tai Chi can help some patients. Discuss with your provider what forms of exercise are appropriate for you.
- Maintain a balanced and healthy diet, including eight 8-ounce glasses of fluid a day and a variety of foods providing protein and carbohydrates, as well as fruits and vegetables.
- Listen to your body. Plan rest periods or a short nap around fatigue or before a social outing.
- Begin a bedtime routine of bathing or listening to music to help you relax and fall asleep faster, as well as sleeping for 8 hours per night.
- Make a plan to feel less tired by letting others help you, doing

important activities first and earlier in the day or taking time off from your job if needed.

Peripheral Neuropathy

Some types of chemotherapy are known to affect the nerves outside the brain. *Peripheral neuropathy* is a general term used to describe changes in peripheral nerves and is a common side effect experienced in patients receiving chemotherapy agents, such as cisplatin and paclitaxel (see table 4.11). Several types of peripheral nerves that can be damaged by chemotherapy: (1) sensory nerves (related to the sense of touch), (2) motor nerves (related to movement and muscle tone), and (3) autonomic nerves (related to involuntary bodily movement, like digestion). Patients who have a history of diabetes, alcohol abuse, or vitamin deficiency are at greatest risk for peripheral neuropathy.

Peripheral neuropathy associated with chemotherapy usually affects the peripheral nerves in the toes, feet, fingers, and hands. Many patients describe the sensation as a tingling, numbness, weakness, burning, or the feeling of "pins and needles" in the fingers or toes, or both. The pattern is generally called "stocking-glove" because the sensation usually does not go above the ankles (stocking) or wrist (glove). The discomfort associated with peripheral neuropathy may cause feelings of imbalance, dizziness, shakiness, trembling, sore muscles, and difficulty with fine motor skills such as writing or buttoning buttons. Walking may be uncoordinated, and simple tasks such as driving may be difficult due to heaviness in the legs and feet.

Although peripheral neuropathy is not life threatening, it can certainly affect an individual's quality of life. The neuropathy is usually

TABLE 4.11   *Chemotherapy Used in Ovarian Cancer That Increases the Risk for Peripheral Neuropathy*

Platinum compounds (cisplatin, carboplatin, oxaliplatin)	Altretamine (Hexalen)
	Thalidomide
Taxanes (docetaxel, paclitaxel)	Vinorelbine (Navelbine)*
Vincristine (Oncovin)	

*To a lesser degree than the others.

temporary, although regeneration of nerves is a long process. Symptoms may last up to a year after treatment is completed and in some cases may be permanent. It is important to report any symptoms of peripheral neuropathy to your provider, as symptoms may continue to worsen throughout treatment. The dose of your treatment may be reduced to prevent long-term peripheral neuropathy. A number of drugs, such as amifostine, glutathione, and vitamin E, have been evaluated as prevention strategies for peripheral neuropathy and have shown no demonstrated effect. Calcium and magnesium supplements have been shown to prevent peripheral neuropathy but are not widely used due to concerns related to decreasing the chemotherapy's effectiveness.

Patient Education for Peripheral Neuropathy

- Inform your doctor or nurse immediately if you experience any numbness or tingling in your fingers or toes.
- Maintain a safe environment to prevent falls and injury:
  - Wear sturdy and well-fitted shoes that do not easily slip off your feet.
  - Turn the light on before entering a room.
  - Use handrails and a cane for assistance with walking.
  - Cover floors and tubs with nonskid rugs and bath mats.
  - Use rubber gloves and pot holders to protect your hands in the kitchen.
  - Use gloves for gardening.
  - Ask a family member to test the water temperature before you bathe.
- Your doctor or nurse may recommend vitamin B, glutamine powder, or other dietary supplements during chemotherapy, although there is not a lot of evidence supporting the effectiveness of these agents in preventing or treating neuropathy.
- Complementary therapies, such as massage, range-of-motion exercises (for example, opening and closing hands), acupuncture, and physical therapy may help with the pain associated with peripheral neuropathy.
- Wearing socks and gloves may relieve discomfort.

- Applying ice or soaking your hands or feet in warm water may provide temporary relief.
- Talk with your doctor about the following medications that may decrease the effects of the burning or tingling:
  - non-narcotic analgesics
  - narcotic analgesics
  - steroids
  - antiepileptic drugs
  - antidepressants
  - topical numbing creams
- Talk with your doctor or nurse about complementary or integrative therapies that may be helpful in reducing the symptoms:
  - transcutaneous electric nerve stimulation (TENS)
  - acupuncture or acupressure
  - therapeutic massage
  - yoga or Tai Chi
- Talk with your doctor or nurse about getting a referral to physical and occupational therapy for an exercise program and assistive devices to make activities of daily living easier.

Memory Changes (Cognitive Function)

Chemotherapy can injure the central nervous system (CNS), the part of the brain that coordinates muscle movement, reflexes, and thinking. Although women who have received chemotherapy have reported subtle changes in cognitive function or memory loss, these symptoms have in the past been overlooked. But that is true no longer. Among patients in support groups and networking classes, these memory changes from chemotherapy are affectionately referred to as "chemo-brain." Changes in memory, concentration, and language skills can occur up to two years after chemotherapy has been completed. These changes can be distressing for individuals and family members. Many patients are worried that something is seriously wrong, such as a brain tumor or Alzheimer disease. It is important to report any such symptoms to your doctor to determine the cause.

Besides chemotherapy, many other factors can affect concentration and memory: stress, anxiety, depression, and other medications. There are, however, specific chemotherapy agents that place the individual at increased risk for central nervous system toxicity. Toxicity generally occurs while the patient is receiving chemotherapy but may continue after treatment is completed. Report any of the following symptoms immediately to your doctor or nurse: blurred vision, slurred speech, difficulty walking, confusion, or seizures. Ifosfamide is a chemotherapy agent that is often associated with CNS changes. In addition, fluorouracil may also cause CNS changes; however, these side effects are less common. Sometimes chemotherapy with these drugs must be stopped if CNS changes are severe.

Patient Education for "Chemo-Brain"

- Inform your doctor or nurse of any memory changes, muscle weakness, and feelings of confusion, sadness, or depression.
- Keep a to-do list or record things important to remember to help plan and organize your activities.
- Complete important tasks that require thinking at those times in the day when you feel best.
- Write down questions you have for your doctor or nurse, and bring the list with you to your appointment.
- Bring a tape recorder to appointments if you have trouble remembering what has been said.
- Use a pill box or calendar to monitor your prescribed medication.
- Reduce the stress in your life that you can control.
- Be sure to get extra rest.
- Play word games to keep your brain exercising.
- Ask for extra help from friends or family when you need it.

Hand-Foot Syndrome (Palmar-Plantar Erythrodysesthesia)

Hand-foot syndrome (known as *palmar-plantar erythrodysesthesia*, or PPE) is a condition in which the palms of the hands and the soles of the feet become red and dry, peel, and form blisters. Patients describe the skin sensations as anything from burning, with or without swelling, to severe pain. The cause is poorly understood. This condition may affect a patient's quality of life and psychological well-being. Several chemotherapy agents increase the risk of this side effect. The agents most commonly associated with hand-foot syndrome are fluorouracil, liposomal doxorubicin, and capecitabine (see table 4.12). Although hand-foot symptoms are not life threatening, they may interfere with daily activities, and chemotherapy may be delayed or stopped if the reaction is severe. The risk of PPE is increased in elderly patients receiving chemotherapy, because the outer layers of their skin are more fragile. In addition, women are more likely to experience PPE than men, perhaps due to slower metabolism and circulatory systems.

Hand-foot syndrome may appear after the first cycle of chemotherapy and persist or get worse throughout treatment. Although patients may not report it until it becomes severe or uncomfortable, you should inform your doctor or nurse even if the symptoms are not bothersome or severe, such as redness or tingling of hands or feet. It's a good idea to avoid direct sunlight for the first three days after receiving a chemotherapy known to cause PPE and to wear loose clothing and socks and shoes that are not too tight and that do not cause pressure. Taking pyridoxine (vitamin B_6), cyclo-oxygenase-2 (COX-2) inhibitors, or oral corticosteroids may be effective in preventing and treating PPE and should be discussed with your provider. Other soothing remedies are moisturizing creams and lotions applied to your hands and feet. Bag Balm is a petroleum-jelly-like lotion that is recommended for the feet. Many patients put on socks after applying Bag Balm.

TABLE 4.12   *Chemotherapy Used in Ovarian Cancer That Increases the Risk for Hand-Foot Syndrome*

Fluorouracil (5-FU)
Liposomal doxorubicin (Doxil)
Capecitabine (Xeloda)

Patient Education for Hand-Foot Syndrome

- Inform your doctor or nurse of any symptoms of hand-foot syndrome. These include redness of the skin, tingling, burning, swelling, or pain or tenderness on the palms of your hands or the soles of your feet.
- Use moisturizing creams and lotions on your feet and hands daily.
- Ask your doctor or nurse about taking vitamin B_6, COX-2 inhibitors, or oral corticosteroids to prevent or reduce the severity of hand-foot syndrome.
- Avoid direct sunlight for three days after receiving any chemotherapy known to cause hand-foot syndrome. Use sunscreen (SPF 15 or higher) at all times when you are out in the sunlight.
- Avoid tight-fitting clothes, restrictive undergarments, tight elastic waist- or wristbands, or any activity that causes friction for about a week after receiving any chemotherapy agent that causes hand-foot syndrome.
- Avoid skin exposure to heat or hot water, as this can worsen hand-foot syndrome.
- Wear shoes and socks that are properly fitted and that do not cause pressure, rubbing, or blisters. Avoid strappy sandals or high heels that may put pressure on areas of your feet. Jogging, aerobics, jumping, or long walks may make symptoms of PPE worse.
- Avoid putting pressure on bony areas of your body (avoid kneeling and leaning on your elbows).
- Apply ice packs to your hands and feet to provide comfort and constriction of the blood vessels in your extremities. Alternate ice packs on and off every 20 minutes.

Infusion Reactions

Reactions to chemotherapy can occur with almost any drug used to treat cancer and can be defined as any unexpected reaction unknown as a common drug side effect. Chemotherapy-induced infusion reactions can occur immediately at the beginning of the infusion or at any time as a result of repeated exposure to the drug. Infusion reactions may be true allergic reactions, or they may be more related to an immune response. Regardless of the mechanism behind the reaction, the symptoms may be mild or severe and can frighten both patients and families when they occur.

Mild to moderate infusion reactions may produce symptoms such as flushing, rash, fever, rigors, chills, shortness of breath, or low blood pressure. Severe infusion reactions may be associated with spasms in the chest that cause coughing, wheezing, hives, swelling of the airway, low blood pressure that requires treatment, changes in heartbeat, unconsciousness, seizure, abdominal cramping and pain, and abrupt vomiting. Although these symptoms seem scary, your infusion nurse will monitor you closely before, during, and for a period after your chemotherapy infusion to ensure your safety and prompt treatment of any infusion reactions.

Some chemotherapy agents are known to cause reactions, such as cisplatin, carboplatin, oxaliplatin, paclitaxel, and monoclonal antibodies, and your doctor or nurse will give you appropriate medications prior to the infusion to prevent such a reaction. These pre-medications often include antihistamines and corticosteroids and greatly reduce the incidence of infusion reactions. Your provider and nurse will ask you questions about your past medical history and prior drug allergies to further reduce your risk of reaction to the chemotherapy. Before giving your chemotherapy, your infusion nurse will provide you with information on common early symptoms of an infusion reaction. In addition, your vital signs will be taken frequently during the infusion to identify and treat any symptoms of an infusion reaction early.

You need to immediately report any unusual feelings during your chemotherapy infusion to your nurse. If your nurse suspects an infusion reaction, he or she will stop the medication immediately and stay with you to monitor your vital signs. It is very important to remain as calm as possible and remember that most infusion reactions are mild and produce no harm to the patient. Patients experiencing infusion reactions may need additional medications to help relieve symptoms experienced during the reaction. Many patients who experience infusion reactions are safely "re-challenged" with the chemotherapy medication. Other supportive medications are added that make it possible for many patients not to have problems in future treatments with the same medication that caused problems previously.

Patient Education for Infusion Reactions

- Discuss with your provider the likelihood of an infusion reaction to your specific chemotherapy agent.
- Review the symptoms of a typical infusion reaction with your doctor and nurse prior to starting your chemotherapy.
- Ask your doctor if there is a need for pre-medication before your chemotherapy to prevent infusion reaction and be sure to take the medication as directed.
- Give an accurate medical and drug allergy history to all your providers.
- Be sure to notify your nurse immediately if you experience any symptoms of an infusion reaction when your treatment begins.
- Remember to stay calm and breathe deeply if you experience an infusion reaction. Keep reminding yourself that your nurse will take good care of you, and the chances of your being able to continue with treatment are very good.

Conclusion

Every woman's journey with ovarian cancer is personal and unique. Although many women have similar responses to the same treatment, nothing is more important than the individual's own experience and response. In this chapter we have described certain specific side effects of chemotherapy. Other effects and reactions may also occur, depending on individual differences in height, weight, and prior medical history. The primary focus of this chapter has been to describe the more common ailments, to educate you about and make you aware of potential problems so that intervention (and indeed prevention) can be instituted early, before the side effects start or become severe.

Going through chemotherapy is not pleasant or easy. However, improvements continue to be made in managing the side effects of treatment that in years past have caused women to stop treatment prematurely. Recognizing what to expect, when to call your doctor, and how to manage problems when they arise are all important components of your overall treatment program.

You and your health care team need to be partners in your planned care, including recognizing and managing side effects early. Managing the side effects allows effective treatment to be given without interruption or delay, and it increases the potential for maintaining your quality of life while you are having treatment. Collaboration between the patient and the health care team is the most effective strategy for managing chemotherapy side effects and for achieving desirable physical and emotional outcomes, and thus for easing a woman's cancer journey.

CHAPTER 5

Radiation Therapy

Richard Zellars, MD

R adiation has a storied past in the management of ovarian cancer. There are both *retrospective* (analyzing data from events
that have already occurred) and *prospective* (collecting data from
events as they occur) randomized studies showing a benefit with
whole-abdominal radiation compared with pelvic-only radiation or
no radiation at all. The success associated with whole-abdominal
and pelvic radiation, however, was before the era of modern effective
chemotherapy. Since then, although effective, radiation use in this
disease is far more limited.

Whole-Abdominal Radiation

Whole-abdominal radiation has been successfully used in the
management of epithelial ovarian cancer. In randomized trials comparing whole-abdominal radiation to chemotherapy, however, radiation did not result in superior outcomes and was associated with
worse toxicity. These studies were somewhat problematic as they
included patients with advanced-stage disease and did not use what

many would consider modern chemotherapy regimens. Nevertheless, whole-abdominal radiation fell out of favor.

Although not as popular as it once was, interest in whole-abdominal radiation persists. Investigators are exploring modern whole-abdominal radiation techniques with lower doses (which should decrease toxicity) and with radiation-sensitizing drugs. For example, an ongoing study is evaluating the benefit of whole-abdominal radiation with concurrent *poly adenosine diphosphate (ADP) ribose polymerase inhibitors (PARPi)*. PARPi are of great interest in ovarian cancer because preliminary studies have shown that PARPi are an effective treatment in late-stage ovarian cancer. Because PARPi work by inhibiting cancer cells' ability to repair single strand *deoxyribonucleic acid* (DNA) breaks, it makes sense to combine them with radiation, which causes single-strand DNA breaks. PARPi should enhance radiation therapy's efficacy. Although the results of this and other studies reassessing the modern uses of whole-abdominal radiation are years off, one can safely assume that the future of this old technique is still evolving.

Isolated Local Recurrences

Approximately 55 percent of epithelial ovarian cancers recur within the first year after treatment. Unfortunately, it is difficult to achieve long-term survival or cure after a recurrence. Studies have shown that tumors that recur less than six months after chemotherapy are likely to be resistant to chemotherapy (*chemo-resistant*). It is perhaps in this situation that radiation is most useful. Radiation in this group has been shown to result in prolonged progression-free survival and high rates of local (pelvic) control. Those most likely to benefit are women who have (1) an isolated local or loco-regional (pelvic-abdominal) recurrence, (2) a long disease-free interval, and (3) the recurrence completely resected (surgically removed). If the recurrence is limited to a particular site but is not resectable, salvage radiation may still be a valid option. Given recent advances in radiation therapy, *localized radiation* (radiation to one particular site) can be well tolerated with low likelihood of significant toxicity. Women with widespread disease are least likely to benefit.

Intraperitoneal Radiation Therapy

Intraperitoneal (IP) radiation therapy (or radiotherapy) is a way of delivering radiation through the abdominal wall into the peritoneal fluid. It can be delivered via radioactive *colloids* (microscopic particles) or be more directed via radio-labeled antibodies, also known as *radioimmunotherapy* (RIT). These radio-labeled antibodies, or in the case of colloids, particles, are placed in the abdominal cavity, where they deliver a dose of radiation therapy over a short distance to any structure they touch. This would seem ideal to treat the lining of the peritoneal cavity, where micro-metastases may exist. Additionally, this technique limits the dose to the normal intestinal walls and structures. The use of these materials was proposed for women with isolated disease in the ovary or ovaries when, even though the disease had been completely removed, washings in the abdomen had demonstrated the presence of cancer cells (called FIGO Stage IC; see table 2.1 in chapter 2).

Clearly, the success of this technique depends on the free flow of peritoneal fluid throughout the abdominal cavity such that the colloids or radio-labeled antibodies have full access to the peritoneal lining. However, these treatments are delivered after a surgery, which often produces *adhesions* (scar tissue) that limit the flow of the peritoneal fluid. The restricted flow results in large areas of the peritoneal space becoming "sanctuaries," where cancer cells can literally hide from the IP radiotherapy. The sanctuaries that are created may lead to disease recurrence. An additional disadvantage is that IP radiotherapy may cause more adhesions, which limit flow of the peritoneal fluid, complicate future surgeries, and promote bowel obstructions. Given these limitations, IP radiotherapy is rarely used today, although it may be an option for some patients who cannot receive more standard methods of treatment.

Germ Cell Neoplasms

Some malignancies arise from the *germ cells* (the cells that produce the eggs that eventually can be fertilized and lead to the development of an embryo). These malignancies, and particularly the ones called *dysgerminomas,* are exquisitely sensitive to radiation therapy. When these lesions have been surgically removed, and when it is known that the cancer has spread to local lymph nodes, radiation therapy to only that area is a rational choice.

Local radiation therapy is still used to treat dysgerminomas when chemotherapy has failed, when the patient chooses not to use chemotherapy, when the patient's medical condition precludes the use of chemotherapy, or because of other considerations. This treatment has fallen out of favor, however, due to its side effects and because multiagent chemotherapy has been demonstrated to be equally effective in treating dysgerminomas.

Conclusion

Although radiation was once a major treatment in the management of ovarian cancer, improved systemic agents and persistent toxicity with standard radiation have limited its use to patients who are unable to receive, or whose disease recurred after, standard surgery and chemotherapy. Research continues to refine the use of radiation, and it may one day become a valid treatment option in earlier staged patients again.

CHAPTER 6

Nutrition

Ana Milena Angarita Africano, MD, and Amanda Nickles Fader, MD

W estern medicine, and specifically Western medicine as practiced in the United States, tends to assign nutrition a secondary role in the management of malignancies. We firmly believe this approach is misguided at best and can be harmful to patients. It makes sense intuitively to consider adequate nutrition an essential part of treatment along with optimal surgery and chemotherapy, and a growing catalog of scientific data supports this approach. Nutrition, for many health care professions, has long been considered "complementary" therapy, but because proper nutrition improves the outcome of treatment, we treat our patients with nutrition as aggressively as we treat them with surgery and chemotherapy.

In this chapter, we describe how ovarian cancer affects nutrition and how nutritional support can improve the outcome of treatment for ovarian cancer. We also offer suggestions for maintaining a healthy diet during and after treatment.

How Does Ovarian Cancer Affect Nutrition?

Why are women with ovarian cancer malnourished in the first place? There are three basic reasons, and for many women, all three come into play.

First, a woman may have been malnourished before she developed ovarian cancer. Many Americans are amazed that they can be "malnourished" while weighing more than they should! Although this phenomenon is not unique to the United States, we Americans seem to be better at it than anyone else in the world. Left to their own devices, many people eat the wrong things, and too much of them. People who are obese are more likely than not to be malnourished: they have deficiencies in protein and other essential nutrients and vitamins as a result of their high-fat, high-complex-carbohydrate diets. The lean American is more likely to be nutritionally fit and often is more fit from a cardiovascular standpoint as well. But elderly people (and women with ovarian cancer commonly are elderly), particularly if they are poor or have limited financial resources, may be malnourished not only in proteins and other essential nutrients but also in total calorie intake.

Second, a woman may be malnourished because of the ovarian cancer itself. When ovarian cancer spreads outside the ovaries, it often grows on the surface of the intestines and stomach or pushes on these structures. This growth can lead to narrowing and irritation of the intestines and stomach and can interfere with the woman's ability to take in or tolerate oral feedings, making it impossible for her to consume adequate calories and obtain necessary nutrients.

Finally, even a woman who is eating normally and healthily may become malnourished because the ovarian cancer consumes large amounts of calories and nutrients. Anything that is growing (like Rick's son Jake when he was 10 years old) or that is metabolically very active (like his adult son Rob, when he was long-distance running) burns more calories than something that is not growing or not active. Ovarian cancer is both growing and very biologically active. Therefore, simply having ovarian cancer is a nutritional drain on the body.

How Does Nutrition Affect Treatment for Ovarian Cancer?

We have established why nutritional deficiencies are common in women with ovarian cancer. Now, what is the "cost" to the patient of these deficiencies?

Nutrition and Major Surgery

For centuries, surgeons have realized that malnourished patients are more likely to have complications following major surgery and are less likely to survive the operation. Malnutrition affects recovery from surgery in two basic ways: (1) impaired healing of the surgical site, whether the site of a bowel anastomosis (reconnection) or a site on the anterior (front) abdominal wall, and (2) the ability to resist and fight infection.

Wound healing

For a surgical site to heal quickly and securely, the body must contain adequate amounts of essential protein, vitamins, and trace elements at the time of surgery. Many women with ovarian cancer, particularly if there has been a delay in the diagnosis and treatment of the malignancy, will have had some degree of intestinal dysfunction, as discussed earlier, causing a decrease in the intake of necessary nutrition. There may also be underlying issues of malnutrition associated with existing but unrelated medical problems such as diabetes, obesity (remember that many obese women are actually protein deficient), irritable or inflammatory bowel disease, and so on. Inadequate nutrition often leads to an increased possibility of wound separation, hernias, failure of intestinal anastomosis, and other problems.

Resisting and fighting infection

The human body cannot resist and fight infection as well when it has nutritional deficiencies as it does when it is well nourished. Because women who are having major surgical debulking procedures for ovarian cancer are undergoing a surgery that, although "clean," is commonly "contaminated" with bacteria, any failure in the body's ability to fight infections can be disastrous.

It's easy to see that the nutritional situation at the time of making the abdominal wall incision is extremely important. To improve a patient's nutritional well-being and increase the probability of a successful surgical outcome, it is recommended that a short period (about ten days) of intense nutritional supplementation be administered through intravenous feeding, either *total parenteral nutrition* (TPN) or *partial parenteral nutrition* (PPN). *Parenteral* refers to the fact that the nutritional supplementation is bypassing the intestinal (enteral) tract (see below). We often delay surgery or chemotherapy to improve nutrition in women who are markedly nutritionally impaired.

Immune Function during Chemotherapy

The immune function is the body's mechanism to identify anything that is different, or foreign, and to kill it and clear it from the body. Maximal immune function is imperative for maximal cancer cell destruction. Because most chemotherapeutic regimens used to treat ovarian cancer lead to a decrease in the number of white blood cells (the cells that fight infection), it is essential for the white cells that *are* circulating to work as well as they can. Patients who are nutritionally impaired are more likely to have white cells that don't work as well at finding things that need to be killed and at killing them and clearing them from the body. In someone who is malnourished and undergoing chemotherapy, an impaired immune system can lead to less effective chemotherapy as well as an increased risk of infection and reduced ability to fight infection.

Achieving and Preserving Adequate Nutrition

As noted at the beginning of this chapter, we are as aggressive in nutritionally treating women with ovarian cancer as we are with our use of surgery and chemotherapy. For women with documented major nutritional abnormalities who are not able to consistently take in adequate oral nutrition (as shown by formal assessment during their hospitalization), we provide parenteral nutritional support until they have nutritionally "healed" and have demonstrated that they can receive adequate oral nutrition consistently. For many women, nutritional treatment is required for many weeks if not months as the patient's nutritional deficit is corrected, and the tumor load is decreased.

For a woman who does not have a nutritional deficiency at the time of diagnosis and initiation of therapy for ovarian cancer, everything possible must be done to try to make sure that she remains nutritionally intact during her subsequent chemotherapy. Chemotherapy has numerous side effects, and the management of these side effects is complex.

It is often difficult for a woman undergoing multiagent chemotherapy to maintain adequate caloric and nutritional intake. This difficulty can be the result of gastrointestinal toxicity from the chemotherapy, appetite suppression from medications, and depression associated with the diagnosis of ovarian cancer, among other causes. Regardless of the cause or causes, a proactive approach must be taken to ensure that she does not develop a nutritional abnormality.

So far in this chapter, we have discussed the very important topic of nutrition in women with ovarian cancer: how nutrition can be adversely affected by ovarian cancer and its treatment and why it is so important to maintain good nutrition. In the rest of the chapter, we provide more specific information about nutritional needs and sources of nutrition that can be used as a woman is returning (it is hoped) to her pre-ovarian-cancer state.

Nutrition during Chemotherapy

For most women, eating a well-balanced diet that includes plenty of fruits, vegetables, and whole-grain products as well as a moderate amount of protein (low-fat meat) and dairy products is usually not difficult. For the reasons discussed earlier, however, ovarian cancer treatment and the side effects of treatment can compromise a woman's ability to consume a healthy diet. The specific side effects of treatment vary, depending on the chemotherapy drugs that are administered, although certain side effects are experienced by almost everyone to some degree.

The most common side effects of ovarian cancer chemotherapy treatment that may affect a woman's nutritional status are nausea, vomiting, loss of appetite, and a change in the sense of taste or smell. Diarrhea and constipation may also occur, although they are less common. Chemotherapy can lead to a general sense of fatigue, sometimes meaning you are just too tired to prepare and eat a proper meal. Rarely, chemotherapy treatments can cause sores to form in the mouth and throat and make it physically painful to swallow food or liquid; this situation can lead to malnutrition and dehydration.

Although these side effects are time limited (they will go away after treatment is completed), they can make it very difficult to maintain your strength during therapy. To help maintain your strength during chemotherapy, we suggest you follow some or all of the following suggestions.

Maintain a positive attitude

Maintaining a positive attitude is critical to the process of surviving ovarian cancer. Take a positive attitude about improving your overall health and your body's ability to get through treatment by attending to your nutritional needs and maintaining your strength. Be proactive about deciding what you put in your body. Focus on seeing nutrition, along with exercise and getting plenty of sleep, as an important part of a healthy lifestyle, which is conducive to maintaining a positive attitude.

Develop a nutritional plan

We always recommend that before beginning chemotherapy treatment, patients have a formal consultation with an experienced dietitian or nutritionist to develop an individual nutritional plan or program. These professionals are familiar with how cancer treatment can affect nutritional intake and will design a dietary regimen based on your personal likes and dislikes that still satisfies your nutritional needs. Eating is much easier if you are eating foods that you like, even if it means eating for dinner what you would normally eat for breakfast.

It is important to include foods with high caloric and nutritional value, especially those that contain potassium, calcium, iron, and magnesium, as these foods will help your body recover from surgery and alleviate some of the side effects of chemotherapy. Supplementing meals with nutritious snacks can be a good source of extra calories and protein (see table 6.1). Try to keep a variety of snacks on hand that you can eat during the day and that are easy to prepare. Suggestions include soup, cereal and milk, yogurt, and half a sandwich. Be careful to avoid snacks that might make the side effects of chemotherapy treatment worse (for example, don't eat large amounts of fruits and raw vegetables if you are having diarrhea). Our patients have found it helpful to meet with their dietitian periodically throughout the course of treatment, to review how their nutritional program is working for them and make any necessary adjustments.

Plan ahead

After you have developed your nutritional plan, spend some time thinking about what foods you will need a week or two in advance. Stock up on food products while you are feeling well enough to go shopping (don't wait until right after a treatment, when fatigue will be the most noticeable). It is also a good idea to prepare some of your meals in advance, so you won't have to do as much cooking immediately after each treatment.

Make use of all your resources

Don't be afraid to ask your family and friends to help you with your nutritional program. They can shop for you and prepare foods and meals. Family and friends are usually anxious and willing to participate in your care. Helping with shopping and cooking is a great way to get them directly involved and give them the satisfaction of knowing that they are actively helping you to get better and stronger.

Make sure you are obtaining the necessary nutrients

Side effects of treatment, such as persistent nausea or mouth sores, can prevent you from consuming adequate calories. In addition, ovarian cancer itself can cause problems, such as a partial bowel obstruction, that make it difficult to stay adequately nourished. Although not ideal, there are several alternatives to eating by mouth in these circumstances.

A *gastric feeding tube* is a thin, flexible tube that is placed directly

TABLE 6.1 *American Cancer Society Nutritional Recommendations for Ovarian Cancer Survivors*

Dietary pattern	• Rich in vegetables and fruits • Whole grain rather than refined grain • Fish and poultry rather than red meat and processed meat • Low-fat rather than full-fat dairy products
For inadequate nutrition	If food is not enough, add fortified, commercially prepared or homemade nutrient-dense beverages or foods
For overweight or obese	Increase physical activity and avoid sugars (honey, brown sugar, high-fructose corn syrup, soft drinks, and fruit-flavored drinks)
Alcohol	Limit to 1 or 2 drinks a day, if any

into the stomach through the abdominal wall. Once in place, high-calorie nutrition formulas can be delivered through the tube. Feeding tubes are used when someone is unable to physically eat but still has a functioning intestinal (digestive) tract. Ideally, oral intake should be resumed as soon as possible.

Parenteral nutrition can be used when there is a serious problem with the digestive tract, such as partial obstruction, severe vomiting, or diarrhea, and adequate nutrients cannot be absorbed from the intestines. Parenteral nutrition involves administering a nutritional solution through the vein (intravenously). Both gastric tube and parenteral nutrition can be given at home.

After Treatment Ends

Most of the side effects of chemotherapy will dissipate within a few weeks of completing the final treatment. If problems such as poor appetite or a change in taste or smell persist longer than this, it is a good idea to talk with your doctor, nurse, or dietitian to develop a plan to address the issue. Weight gain or weight maintenance should be managed with a combination of diet, physical activity, and changes in habits. If you need to gain weight, this means increasing energy intake. If you need to maintain weight, this means reducing caloric intake and increasing energy use through physical activity. Eating well and maintaining good nutritional status after your treatment has ended is an excellent way to regain your strength, rebuild tissue, improve your energy level, and feel better overall.

A Healthy Diet and Ovarian Cancer

A healthy diet remains one of the key lifestyle factors thought to improve response to treatment, improve quality of life, speed recovery, and decrease the risk of a recurrence. In addition, eating a balanced diet aids in the prevention of other chronic diseases that can occur in women who have or who have had ovarian cancer.

Eat a Balanced Diet

There are foods with high-energy density (high number of calories per cup) and with low-energy density (low number of calories per cup). We should reduce the energy density of the diet by eating more low-energy-dense foods (water and fiber-rich vegetables and fruits) and avoiding or at least reducing the portion sizes of the high-energy dense foods (such as cheese). The low-energy-dense foods have the added advantage of making you feel full if you are trying to lose or maintain weight.

- Protein: Eating protein is essential for everyone and is particularly important during all phases of survivorship. You can meet protein needs with foods containing low saturated fats such as fish, lean meat, skinless poultry, eggs, nonfat and low-fat dairy products, and nuts and seeds.
- Carbohydrates: Rich sources are vegetables, fruits, whole grains, and legumes.
- Fiber: Choose whole grains and whole-grain food products over fiber supplements and refined grains. Refined grains (white flour, white bread, white rice) have fewer vitamins and minerals and less fiber than whole grains.

Generally Avoid Supplements

Many cancer experts do not recommend the use of vitamins, minerals, and other dietary supplements such as antioxidants during or after treatment. They suggest that these supplements be used only when a woman has a specific, diagnosed nutrient deficiency. It is reasonable to take a regular multivitamin, but large doses of vitamins, herbs, or other non-FDA-approved supplements during or after surgery or chemotherapy treatment may be harmful to your health and will not improve cancer-related outcomes.

What's Best to Eat?

Whether you want to gain, lose, or maintain weight, experts recommend that cancer survivors follow these guidelines for a healthy diet:

- Eat a minimum of five servings of fruits and vegetables a day. A serving can be a cup of dark leafy greens or berries, a medium fruit, or a half cup of other colorful choices; use plant-based seasonings like parsley and turmeric.
- Go for whole grains. Opt for high-fiber breads and cereals, including brown rice, barley, bulgur, and oats; avoid refined foods such as donuts and white bread as well as foods high in sugar.
- Choose lean protein. Stick to fish, poultry, and tofu, limiting red meat and processed meats.
- Keep dairy low fat. Select skim milk, low-fat yogurt, and reduced-fat cheeses.

Other tips to maximize nutrition:

- Aim for a variety of foods. Create a balanced plate that is one-half cooked or raw vegetables, one-fourth lean protein (chicken, fish, lean meat, or dairy), and one-fourth whole grains.
- Eat fatty fish, such as salmon, sardines, and canned tuna, at least twice a week. The fats in these fish are the "good"

heart-healthy omega-3 fats; other sources of these fats include walnuts, canola oil, and flaxseeds.

- Limit alcohol consumption. Alcohol has been linked to cancer risk. Women should have no more than one or two drinks a day, if any.
- Eat foods high in vitamin D. These include salmon, sardines, fortified orange juice, fortified milk, and fortified cereal. Although the optimal intake of calcium and vitamin D is uncertain, in 2010, the Institute of Medicine released a report on dietary intake requirements for calcium and vita-min D. Its Recommended Dietary Allowance (RDA) of vitamin D for children 1 to 18 years and adults through age 70 years is 600 international units (15mcg) daily. Its RDA is 800 inter-national units (20mcg) daily after age 71 years. The intake can be provided in the diet or as a vitamin D supplement. For older adults and those with limited sun exposure, the recommendation is for supplementation with 600 to 800 international units of vitamin D daily. You might ask your physician whether you should have a blood test to measure vitamin D levels.
- Eat foods high in calcium (but low fat). Dairy products have the highest calcium content per serving. In postmenopausal women with osteoporosis, 1,200mg of calcium daily (total diet plus supplement) and 800 international units of vitamin D daily are advised by the Institute of Medicine. Although the optimal intake (diet plus supplement) has not been clearly established in premenopausal women or in men with osteo-porosis, 1,000mg of calcium (total of diet and supplement) and 600 international units of vitamin D daily are generally suggested. Optimal intake can be achieved with a combina-tion of diet plus supplements, but preference is that at least half comes from dietary sources.
- Food—not supplements—is the best source of vitamins and minerals. There is no evidence that dietary supplements provide the same anticancer benefits as fruits and vegetables, and some high-dose supplements may actually increase cancer risk.

- Be "mindful" when eating: this means looking at your food, paying attention to what you are eating, and eliminating or filtering out distractions such as television news. Research suggests that we tend to eat more calories and food with fewer nutrients when we are watching TV, driving, or doing other activities.
- Organic or not? Research on the nutritional benefits of organic fruits and vegetables has been mixed, and no studies have examined whether organic produce is better at preventing cancer or cancer recurrence than nonorganic produce. You should buy whatever produce you like and rinse all fruits and vegetables thoroughly with clean water. Buying or not buying organic foods is a personal choice. For more information on pesticides in produce, visit the Environmental Working Group's Shopper's Guide at ewg.org/foodnews.

Incorporating healthier habits into your lifestyle can make you feel better and improve your quality of life after the diagnosis of ovarian cancer.

CHAPTER 7

Controlling Pain and Suffering

Edward Tanner, MD

P ain and suffering are two very different processes, although many people—health care professionals included—often inaccurately equate the two. In this chapter, we discuss these two different but related processes separately, just as we believe they need to be managed separately.

Dealing with Pain

In the 1980s the experts at the Memorial Sloan-Kettering Cancer Center in New York City championed the development of an objective measure of pain, which they called the fifth vital sign. (The other four vital signs are temperature, heart rate, breathing rate, and blood pressure.) The formalization of pain as a vital sign was a great incentive to develop a *linear analogue scale measure of pain,* a well-validated and easy-to-reproduce way of measuring patient discomfort. The pain assessment tool used at the Johns Hopkins Medical Institutions is a 10-point scale that allows patients to either assign a numerical value to their pain or relate their discomfort on a visual scale corresponding to the numerical values.

The formal acceptance of pain as the fifth vital sign means that whenever a patient reports pain or is receiving pain medications, the health care provider needs to measure the patient's pain level often and objectively, using a pain scale instrument. We do this as part of our routine care with every visit that a patient makes to our office, and we store the data as part of the patient's medical record. This allows us to routinely reassess how severe a patient's pain is and whether there has been any change over time.

It is commonly said that simply admitting a problem exists is the most important step in solving it. Sadly, that's not always true. Although we now have a great way to measure pain, health care professionals continue to struggle with providing adequate pain relief for all patients. We are not solely to blame for this problem, though. Even when health care professionals are able to provide adequate pain relief, some patients have difficulty with or refuse to comply with our pain control recommendations.

Why don't patients have adequate pain control? Not surprisingly, there are a number of reasons. Some of these barriers to adequate pain control are legitimate, but the majority can be overcome. In the following list, we consider only the first two to be legitimate barriers to adequate pain control.

1 Patients' intolerance of side effects of pain medications.
2 Patients' inability to afford pain medications.
3 Health care professionals' ignorance about how to control complex and severe pain.
4 Health care professionals' unwillingness to administer adequate drugs because of fear that the patient will become addicted.
5 Patients' unwillingness to take adequate drugs because of fear of becoming addicted.
6 Patients' inability to understand or comply with the complexity of a pain treatment regimen.

Patients Who Have Trouble Tolerating Side Effects

Side effects of pain medication are a real problem for patients, particularly when the person is being started on relatively high doses of medications. We have two ways to improve patient tolerance. First, we try to increase medication doses in a stepwise fashion. This means changing drug doses one at a time and gradually as well as adding new drugs one at a time, only after maximizing the usefulness of current medications. This approach can help to avoid incorporating too many medications into a patient's treatment plan. If this approach is not followed, it can also be difficult to determine whether new side effects are caused by new medications or by increasing doses of existing ones.

Second, we anticipate side effects. We always explain what kinds of side effects can be expected from a particular medication. Not knowing what sort of side effects can occur and then having something unpleasant happen is an example of how a patient can lose control of a situation—something we actively try to avoid. Anything we can do to help prevent this loss of control is an important way to prevent both pain and suffering. This also allows our patients to be active participants in their care. If side effects are encountered, a well-informed patient may be able to more readily let her physician know when they occur so that interventions can be initiated more rapidly. This communication is an important part of the doctor-patient relationship, because early recognition of side effects can allow for earlier interventions, helping to prevent more serious problems. Early recognition is important, and so are preventive treatment strategies against side effects. In many cases, physicians can minimize or prevent side effects entirely with preventive or early intervention.

A classic example of a side effect related to narcotic administration that can be anticipated and minimized is constipation. The majority of patients taking narcotic pain medications will have some degree of constipation. We start all our patients who are taking narcotics on stool softeners and bulking agents. In addition, we stress the importance of dietary changes to address constipation. This includes drinking plenty of noncaffeinated liquids (eight 8-ounce glasses each day at a minimum) and eating bulky foods, such as whole grains, fresh fruits, and vegetables. Foods on the BRAT diet (bananas, rice, applesauce, and toast) or anything "white" (such as white bread, white rice, and white potatoes) should be avoided. Some patients develop constipation despite these strategies. Patients should then call their doctor's office, so the doctor can recommend more aggressive therapies such as enemas or stronger laxatives (polyethylene glycol or lactulose) to help patients avoid an office visit or hospitalization to treat constipation.

Patients Who Cannot Afford Pain Medications

Unfortunately, not being able to afford pain medications is still a common reality for women who have ovarian cancer. Although the Affordable Care Act should in theory provide a greater proportion of patients with adequate health care coverage in the United States, the system is not perfect, and there are gaps in coverage. Even many patients who have adequate overall medical insurance continue to lack robust prescription drug benefits to cover the costs of cancer therapies.

Medicare is a common primary insurer for American women with ovarian cancer. Although prescription drug coverage is better in the Medicare setting, many of our patients are retired and live on a limited income. Considering the high cost of one drug prescription—let alone several prescriptions—it is evident that the cost of prescriptions for someone with ovarian cancer can be a big hit on a limited budget even if the patient is only responsible for a portion of the total cost. Fortunately, many of the pharmaceutical companies have programs for supplying subsidized medications. A great deal of paperwork must still be completed to obtain these benefits. We believe that more work still needs to be done to ensure that all patients receive adequate health care insurance coverage and prescription drug insurance coverage so they can receive comprehensive care.

Health Care Professionals Who Don't Know How to Control Complex and Severe Pain

Pain associated with recurrent malignancies can be some of the most difficult pain to manage. Malignancies of the female genital tract (cervix) and elsewhere (lung and breast) can present a challenge for achieving adequate pain control. Fortunately for most women who have ovarian cancer, the pain associated with the treatment of the disease (especially surgical) can usually be controlled using straightforward and well-tolerated treatment strategies. Even for women with recurrent ovarian cancer nearing the end of life, most do not usually have pain that is difficult to control.

The optimal management of any but the lowest level of pain is outlined in the "Triad of Treatment":

1 Narcotics
   • Short acting
   • Long acting
2 Anti-inflammatories
3 Potentiators
   • Neuroleptics
   • Antidepressants
   • Antianxiety agents
   • Others

Narcotics

Although narcotics are the leading edge of the triad, their use is not well understood by the layperson or even by some clinicians. On one hand, narcotic medications can be very fast acting and last only a short time, such as can be the case with elixirs and intravenous formulations. These drugs have *half-lives* (how long a meaningful circulating level of the drug is in the bloodstream) of only a few minutes. On the other hand, some narcotic medications take hours or days to reach their maximal effect and have a long-lasting half-life, as can be the case with long-acting narcotic pills or transdermal delivery systems (see table 7.1).

TABLE 7.1 *Half-Lives and Side Effects of Common Narcotic Pain Medications*

Medication	Half-Life (hours)	Side Effects
Codeine	2 to 3	Drowsiness, dizziness, confusion, constipation
Oxycodone*	2 to 3	Drowsiness, dizziness, confusion, constipation, nausea and vomiting
Morphine*	2 to 3	Drowsiness, dizziness, confusion, headache, constipation, nausea and vomiting, itching
Hydromorphone	2 to 3	Drowsiness, confusion, headache, flushing, low blood pressure, palpitations, nausea and vomiting, stomach cramps
Levorphanol	12 to 15	Drowsiness, confusion, headache, flushing, low blood pressure, palpitations, itching, nausea and vomiting, stomach cramps
Fentanyl (transdermal)†		Drowsiness, confusion, low blood pressure, slow heart rate, nausea and vomiting, constipation

*Long-acting formulations of oxycodone (OxyContin) and morphine (MS Contin) are also available for twice-daily oral dosing.

†Transdermal delivery systems have durations of 48 to 72 hours.

There are some general rules that we follow when prescribing narcotic pain medications that the layperson should be aware of:

First, we start with a narcotic pain medication that lasts about 4 to 6 hours. If a patient needs to take her pain medication more frequently than that, she should either receive a higher dose of the intermediate-acting medication or be started on a longer-acting medication. In addition, we will often add a non-narcotic pain medication to the initial narcotic (or vice versa), with excellent relief in most cases. This approach can limit the side effects of the narcotic medication that would otherwise be experienced with increasing doses.

Second, severe, or *aggressive,* pain needs aggressive treatment. Although it is important to increase narcotic medications in an appropriate stepwise way (adding about 30 percent of relative analgesic effect with each change), these changes can be made frequently (every 72 hours, more or less, depending upon which medication is used). Furthermore, the addition of a long-acting narcotic can be effective at controlling pain when large doses are required. Although the specifics of how and when these medications should be considered are beyond the scope of this book, we generally try to include the majority of the narcotic dose (70 to 80 percent of the complete dose) in a long-acting formulation in patients with severe chronic pain. This prevents the kinds of peaks and valleys of pain control seen with short-acting narcotics in patients with severe pain. The remaining 20 to 30 percent of the narcotic dose is provided in a short-acting formulation for breakthrough pain, which allows the patient to have some control over her pain medication administration and generally provides better relief than the sole use of short-acting pain medications in the setting of severe pain.

Anti-inflammatories

As alluded to earlier, *nonsteroidal anti-inflammatory drugs* (NSAIDs; see table 7.2) are valuable additions to narcotic pain medications and can also be substituted for narcotic pain medications in some situations. We start almost all our postoperative patients on a long-acting, nonsteroidal anti-inflammatory agent as soon as they are taking any meaningful amount of liquids or solids orally. The early use of NSAIDs has been repeatedly demonstrated to decrease the total amount of narcotic pain medication necessary to obtain adequate pain control, therefore decreasing many of the unpleasant side effects of narcotic pain medications.

Similarly, as soon as it becomes clear that a patient is going to require long-term pain medications, we will add NSAIDs to the pain medication regimen whether or not she is in the postoperative period. *Steroidal* anti-inflammatory medications are not used as part of pain control, simply because the side effects (toxicity) of these medications are quite serious. The risk-benefit ratio, except in certain unique acute settings, is just too high.

Potentiators

The potentiators include a wide variety of drugs, many of which act by preventing the transmission of pain signals by nerves. Others may have a more central action, serving as an antidepressant or antianxiety medication (see table 7.3). Every expert has a preference

TABLE 7.2   *Half-Lives and Side Effects of Common NSAID Pain Medications*

Medication	Half-Life (hours)	Side Effects
Aspirin	3 to 12	Bleeding, low blood pressure, confusion, nausea, heartburn, stomach ulcers, rash
Acetaminophen	3 to 4	Low blood counts, kidney damage
Ibuprofen	3 to 4	Headache, fatigue, itching, rash, vomiting, stomach ulcers, heartburn, diarrhea, constipation
Indomethacin	4 to 5	Headache, dizziness, nausea, constipation, stomach cramps, bleeding
Ketorolac	4 to 7	Edema, headache, dizziness, stomach pain, diarrhea, rash

among the potentiator drugs, but selecting a medication depends in great part upon the type and location of the patient's pain and what other medications she may need. For this reason, the choice of potentiator varies from patient to patient. In general, we will first add a neuroleptic medication (such as gabapentin [Neurontin]) and an anxiolytic (antianxiety) agent (such as lorazepam [Ativan]) to the regimen of short-acting and long-acting narcotics and NSAIDs. Other options include antidepressants (venlafaxine [Effexor] or a similar drug) or a

TABLE 7.3   *Side Effects of Common Potentiator Pain Medications*

Medication	Side Effects
Antidepressants	
Amitriptyline	Restlessness, dizziness, insomnia, rash, weight gain, constipation
Paroxetine	Headache, dizziness, nausea, constipation, diarrhea, low blood pressure
Venlafaxine	Headache, dizziness, somnolence, insomnia, nausea, constipation, anorexia, weakness, rash
Neuroleptics	
Gabapentin	Drowsiness, dizziness, fatigue, edema, nausea and vomiting, itching
Antianxiety agents	
Lorazepam	Sedation, low blood pressure, headache, nausea, rash, nasal congestion

combination of all of the above. Even though this may mean that a patient is taking five different medications to control her pain, the inconvenience of taking multiple medications is offset by the successful control of pain and the improvement in quality of life. As with the use of narcotics, these medications should always be added stepwise to limit toxicity and allow the physician to assess the effect of each drug on the overall picture.

Non-oral means of delivering medications

Other techniques for pain control can be considered in patients who are unable to tolerate oral medications or for whom adequate pain relief just cannot be obtained with conventional means. One option in this setting is the use of a transdermal delivery system, or "pain patch." The patch is worn on the skin and changed every few days to deliver a continuous level of narcotic during that period. More complex regimens involve the use of either *intravenous* (in a vein) or *subcutaneous* (under the skin) infusion systems to deliver narcotics continuously throughout the body. In some cases, a catheter may be inserted into the back (*epidural* or *intrathecal*) so that analgesics can be infused around the nerves to anesthetize them and block the transmission of pain sensation. These systems should only be considered when other options have failed, because they generally require invasive procedures for placement and carry higher risk for complications such as severe infections.

Health Care Professionals Who Are Concerned That the Patient Will Become Addicted

Any number of misunderstandings on the part of health care professionals can interfere with the delivery of optimal patient care. This is one of them. Addiction is both a physiological and a psychological process. Patients who need pain medications to control their discomfort and to allow them to live a life as close to normal as possible do not become "addicted" to the medications that are prescribed.

It's true that over time, patients may need a higher dose of pain medication as they become acclimated to the drugs they are receiving or when disease progresses. Either of these situations may mean that patients require more medication to control more pain. And of course, when medications that have been used for a long time in relatively high doses are stopped, there will be symptoms. Although these symptoms could theoretically be labeled as withdrawal, that is an overstatement. For example, consider people who take a medication to control elevated blood pressure. If they stop taking that medication, their blood pressure will go back up. We don't consider those people as having withdrawal symptoms from their blood pressure medication. Furthermore, they are not addicted to their blood pressure medication—they are merely using it to treat a real medical condition. The same is true of medications to treat cancer pain. *Pain associated with cancer is a disease that deserves treatment, and pain medications are the medically advised best treatment.*

Patients Who Are Afraid of Becoming Addicted

We discussed this issue indirectly in the section above. In our view, doctors and nurses really have an obligation to make sure that patients understand that they will not become addicted but will become healthier if they take pain medications as prescribed. It's worth repeating: pain associated with cancer is a disease that deserves treatment, and pain medications are the medically advised best treatment. Take the pain medications that are recommended to you! If taking pain medication allows you to work, spend time with family, or participate in an activity that is important to you, why deny yourself just to avoid taking pain medication?

Many patients may also have a difficult time confessing to themselves that they are actually having significant amounts of pain. We believe that a lot of patients, though they won't acknowledge it, view the reality that they are having pain as an indication that their cancer is not controlled or is even progressing. In some instances this is true, but in most cases it is not. Doctors and nurses must share with ovarian cancer patients that some degree of pain is a normal part of the recovery from surgery and can be associated with the treatment of cancer. Acknowledging the pain that one is having is not being weak, nor is it accepting "failure." It is being honest with oneself and one's care providers. Enough said.

Patients Who Cannot Understand or Comply with a Pain Treatment Regimen

The therapeutic regimens described earlier in this chapter can be complex, and it may be difficult for patients who are ill or overwhelmed by their diagnosis to process this information. In an effort to keep patients as free from restrictions as possible, doctors generally prescribe oral medications rather than placing them on regimens that are given by non-oral routes, such as intravenous or intramuscular injections.

There are regimens that require fewer oral medications, such as those using a transdermal delivery system (the patch) or an infusion pump. Although the transdermal system can cause local skin irritation, most patients are able to rotate the application site to reduce this effect. Patients who cannot tolerate the patch can use infusion pumps, but these are costly and require skilled assistance in placing the subcutaneous needle, changing the pump, and so on. We have found that with a simplified regimen that is explicitly outlined and printed out for the patient or caregiver, most are able to master the schedules for taking oral medications.

Dealing with Suffering

Suffering is a complex topic, and there is not one single definition. The word *suffering* is defined by the Merriam-Webster dictionary as "pain that is caused by injury, illness, loss, etc.; physical, mental or emotional pain." Others describe suffering as a symptom or process that threatens the patient because of fear, the meaning of the symptom, and concerns about the future. It can be difficult for physicians to make a diagnosis of suffering, especially if they are not constantly considering whether it is occurring. The most important step toward identifying suffering is for the physician to ask the patient whether she is suffering and in what ways. Your physician should be asking you this question, and if he or she does not, you should feel empowered to start the conversation.

Most patients with ovarian cancer will experience suffering at some point during their treatment. Being open with your health care providers about your personal struggles will help them to assist in alleviating your suffering. We know that simply discussing your suffering will not cure the problem, yet we believe that treating suffering is just as important as physically treating your ovarian cancer. We use a multidisciplinary approach, calling on our palliative care colleagues, psychologists, social workers, clergy, and other allied health care professionals to assist us in mitigating your suffering. We break down suffering into four domains: physical, social-relational, psychological, and existential, each domain with its own set of characteristics and methods of intervention to alleviate the suffering.

Physical Suffering

Physical suffering, by definition, includes most of the tangible symptoms experienced by our patients. Physical pain, as discussed above, can cause physical suffering but is far from the only source of suffering for patients with ovarian cancer. Women also face other physical symptoms, sometimes due to the natural course of disease, and in other instances related to treatment. Many patients report instances of suffering from nausea, constipation, general malaise, drowsiness, weakness, neuropathy, and other causes.

In the same way that we have treatment regimens for pain, we also have various modalities to help alleviate other symptoms. If you are experiencing nausea, we will begin by trying to understand the specific cause of your nausea. Sometimes nausea is due to toxins, such as chemotherapy or even opioids that are stimulating an area in your brain that can cause nausea. We may try using medications such as ondansetron (Zofran), prochlorperazine (Compazine), or haloperidol (Haldol). If we think your nausea may be due to slow bowel function, we may suggest a medication that can improve bowel motility, such as metoclopramide (Reglan). There are a large number of antiemetics that each work with a slightly different mechanism. Thus, if one medication isn't working for you, we can try a second, third, or even fourth medication.

Similarly, for constipation we also have a variety of options to use for developing a personalized bowel regimen. We may not be able to "cure" your constipation; however, our goal is to find the best possible balance to allow you to be able to pass stools and remain comfortable. The answer for some patients is to increase the fiber in their diet and increase fluid intake. For others, constipation may be due to difficulties with water balance, and we may recommend using medications such as sorbitol, lactulose, or polyethylene glycol (MiraLax) to increase water in their intestines and minimize hard stools. In patients who may have gut motility problems due to inactivity or narcotic use, we will try senna at bedtime. Last, some patients need additional lubrication to aid the passage of stool and minimize pain. In this case, we will often try docusate, mineral oil, or glycerin suppositories.

Many women experience other forms of physical suffering during treatment for ovarian cancer. In addition to the gynecologic oncologist, other specialists in the medical profession can help control your symptoms. Palliative care is a specialty that focuses on providing patients with relief from symptoms, pain, and the stress of a serious illness. We involve our palliative care specialists not only in the setting of end-of-life care but in any setting where our patients need extra assistance with symptom control.

Social-Relational Suffering

Whatever your life circumstances were before, the diagnosis of ovarian cancer is life changing. Your paradigm shifts. In many cases, long-standing social dynamics are uprooted in an instant. In our experience, the first step to mitigating the effects of these changes is to admit that they exist. Only by acknowledging these changes, can we work to identify ways to limit their effect on our lives.

One of the most obvious changes that occur when a woman is diagnosed with ovarian cancer is the effect the illness can have on living independently. For example, previously simple tasks may be transformed into complex tasks after surgery or during chemotherapy. You may need to rely on your partner to do the laundry or on a friend to take you grocery shopping or to appointments. Many women will find they are dependent on others at times and may feel guilty about the perceived burden they are placing on their support network. This sense of burden is often exaggerated, as family and friends are often more willing to provide assistance than patients realize. By opening up about this feeling of being a burden on family, friends, and the health care team, many patients find that they can rely on more support than anticipated. In addition, your providers may be able to offer strategies to limit the effects of treatment on friends and family. For example, if transportation is a concern, your health care team can often find ways to condense appointments or laboratory tests to limit how often you have to go to the clinic. However, your health care team can only intervene on your behalf if they know about your particular concerns. *Tell them.*

Women with ovarian cancer also struggle in their relationships with loved ones. You may be concerned about how your family is coping with your illness or worry about leaving your loved ones behind. These are normal feelings. If you discuss your concerns with your physicians, they can help you to cope with these struggles and even refer you to appropriate professionals to assist you in meeting your needs. We also encourage all our patients to begin arranging their affairs early on in the treatment course. We hope you will not need these arrangements; however, early planning can help alleviate some stress for both you and your family if you become more ill in the future.

Many individuals diagnosed with ovarian cancer also find that they have new financial concerns. A patient who is the primary breadwinner for her family may worry about her inability to work due to loss of employment or decreased wages. Most patients find that ovarian cancer treatment carries a heavy financial burden: co-pays for hospitalizations and infusion visits, medications, travel costs, and so on all add up over time. Patients without adequate health insurance will be facing even greater challenges. Worrying about financial burdens is another form of real suffering for many of our patients. While we do admit that treatment for ovarian cancer is not cheap, we try to ensure that all our patients have access to proper care. Often, we turn to our social workers, both inpatient and outpatient, to assist with navigating financial barriers. Depending on your specific hospital, there may also be a medical-legal partnership established with a community legal advocate who can assist with legal issues in need of resolution. For financial concerns, this help may come in the form of assistance in applying for Social Security Disability

Insurance, understanding the implications of current rent or mortgage terms, navigating health insurance, and so forth. Resources exist to help you navigate the finances of ovarian cancer.

Psychological Suffering

Depression is a significant symptom in many women with ovarian cancer, and it can be particularly distressing. Too often, symptoms of depression go unrecognized and untreated. In patients who do not have cancer, symptoms associated with depression include loss of energy, fatigue, weight loss, insomnia, difficulty concentrating, and similar problems. Patients with ovarian cancer may experience these symptoms even if they are not clinically depressed. If you are experiencing feelings of hopelessness, worthlessness, guilt, lack of interest where you previously found joy, and sustained periods of feeling sad, you should bring these feelings to the attention of your care team.

For patients who meet the criteria for depression, we again take a multidisciplinary approach to treatment. There are a variety of medication choices at our disposal. For patients who meet the diagnostic criteria of either depression or anxiety disorder, we institute first-line pharmacotherapy. For some patients, especially those closer to the end of life, we may elect to use a psychostimulant, as these medications work quickly. We may use drugs such as dextroamphetamine (Dexedrine), methylphenidate (Ritalin), or pemoline (Cylert). In other situations, we may use standard antidepressant medications, such as the selective serotonin reuptake inhibitors (SSRIs), although these medications can sometimes take up to one month before taking complete effect. In addition to pharmacotherapy, we will also make a referral to our social workers as well as to mental health experts.

Existential Suffering

Women with ovarian cancer will often experience suffering on an existential level. There may be moments when you feel a lack of control, loss of identity, or worry about an unclear future. You may worry about death and dying. Some women feel that they are undergoing a spiritual crisis. These are normal thoughts and concerns women experience while fighting ovarian cancer. Social workers and psychologists can explore these topics in depth with you and your family. For women having a spiritual crisis or who are questioning their faith while in the hospital, chaplains of various faith traditions are available to speak with them. Outside of the hospital, we recommend speaking with your personal pastor, rabbi, or other spiritual adviser, as they have a wealth of knowledge and experience working with congregants during illness and suffering.

For some women, this existential suffering is the most taxing, and we don't want you to have to go through this process on your own.

Throughout this chapter, we hope that you have noticed the most important aspect of dealing with pain and suffering: your physician and health care team are here to help you cope. Although it is our job to explore these issues with you and offer strategies to minimize their impact, we need you to let us know what you are experiencing. Only through this partnership can we have the greatest effect.

CHAPTER 8

Adding Quality to Life

Ramez N. Eskander, MD, and Paula J. Anastasia, RN, MN, AOCN

Despite the aggressive nature of ovarian cancer, advances in treatment and supportive care have translated into improved survival. Specifically, five-year survival rates have steadily improved, rising from 33 percent (between 1975 and 1977) to 44 percent (between 2003 and 2009). Changes in therapy that have been key to this improvement include surgical cytoreduction (removal of all visible cancer at the time of surgery), platinum-based chemotherapy drugs, intraperitoneal chemotherapy (chemotherapy administered directly into the abdominal cavity), novel regimens with weekly administration of chemotherapy, and targeted biologic therapies, including those that target cancer blood vessel growth (*anti-angiogenic therapies*).

As the number of ovarian cancer survivors grows, so does the importance of survivorship care. Too often, treatment of the patient centers on treatment of the cancer, while the effects of interventions such as surgery and chemotherapy on quality of life are ignored. It is for this reason that the Institute of Medicine has promoted the development of evidence-based, comprehensive, compassionate, and coordinated survivorship care plans.

Menopause and Associated Symptoms

One of the most common and distressing side effects that results from removing the ovaries at the time of ovarian cancer surgery is surgically induced menopause. The distress is exceptionally apparent in premenopausal women. A brief review of natural menopause helps explain how surgical menopause affects a patient's quality of life. Traditionally, the menopausal transition lasts four years, with a range anywhere from two to eight years; only a small minority of women (about 10 percent) abruptly stop having menstrual periods. The usual gradual change eases the body's shift to the *hypo-estrogenic* (having less estrogen) state, allowing women to cope with the commonly encountered side effects. The menopausal transition is also often associated with an elevated androgen-to-estrogen ratio, resulting in hirsutism, or excess hair growth in women.

The most commonly associated menopausal symptom is the "hot flash," or "hot flushes," which is a feeling of intense heat with sweating and associated rapid heart rate. Up to 80 percent of women report hot flashes during the menopausal transition. The severity of hot flashes is difficult to predict, and there is significant variation among women. Typically, women experience five to fifteen episodes per day, each lasting 2 to 5 minutes. On average, in natural menopause, these symptoms diminish in one to two years, but they can last up to five years in some women. Biologically, the increase in heart rate and the dilation of small blood vessels that result in the hot flash are caused by a relative activation of the temperature regulatory centers of the brain from the hormonal imbalance induced when the ovaries stop producing estrogen.

Aside from vasomotor symptoms, menopause has been associated with psychophysiological effects, although large-scale studies have failed to demonstrate a definitive link between decreased estrogen levels and depression. Nonetheless, many women report fatigue, nervousness, headaches, insomnia, depression, and irritability as they enter menopause. No direct causation has been identified, but it is hypothesized that hot flashes result in interrupted and fragmented sleep patterns, and that this lack of restorative sleep then translates into the psychological symptoms described above.

The effects of menopause, and lack of estrogen, on cardiovascular health has been debated for many years. The Women's Health Initiative (WHI) was launched in 1991 and consisted of clinical trials designed to test the effects of postmenopausal hormone replacement therapy (HRT) on heart disease, bone fractures, and breast and colorectal cancer. The results reported from the estrogen-plus-progestin (also known as progesterone) component of the study indicated that HRT in this population of patients was associated with an increased risk of heart attack, and the researchers concluded that HRT should not be used to prevent cardiovascular disease. Importantly, however, since that time, critical review of the study findings have resulted in a gradual reassessment of the primary conclusions. The hypothesized impact of HRT on cardiovascular health occurs early in menopause and is related to an effect on cholesterol and lipid profiles. During the menopausal transition, there is an increase in total cholesterol and low-density lipoproteins, resulting in increased cardiovascular risk. In elegant animal studies, it was shown that early initiation of estrogen after surgical removal of the ovaries prevented buildup of atherosclerotic plaques on the coronary blood vessels. These plaques cause a narrowing of the arteries that predisposes a person to heart attacks. Herein lies the primary criticism of the WHI, as the average age of women in the group who were given the estrogen-progestin combination was over 63 years, more than 10 years beyond the average age of menopause in healthy women, meaning that the cardiovascular effect of a hypo-estrogenic (low estrogen) state was already established in these women. As such, it is incorrect to conclude from the WHI study results that HRT increases coronary clinical events (e.g., heart attack) in all women.

Conversely, menopause's direct effect on bone health has been well established. Thirteen to 18 percent of women older than 50 years have osteoporosis (brittle bones), making them more susceptible to fractures and the complications that follow from fractures. The most common sites of osteoporosis include the lumbar spine (lower back), radius (wrist), and femoral neck (hip). Specifically, bone mass declines at a rate of 2 to 5 percent per year for the first five to ten years after menopause, and then at a rate of approximately 1 percent per year thereafter. This results from a decline in estrogen levels and an increased responsiveness to hormones that lead to bone destruction and release of calcium. The administration of estrogen after menopause has been shown to protect against this bone loss.

Last, the effects of menopause on the vagina and vaginal lubrication have been well described. In response to low estrogen levels, the vagina becomes *atrophic* (mean the vaginal tissue thins and shrinks), resulting in inflammation, itching, pain with intercourse, bleeding due to tears in the vaginal lining, and a progressive narrowing of the vaginal canal. These physiological changes are partly a result of an alteration in the normal bacterial flora of the vagina. In addition, the drop in estrogen levels results in decreased vaginal blood flow, and a subsequent decline in vaginal lubrication. These changes directly affect sexual function and can result in significant alterations in perception and body image. In scientific studies, it appears that cancer survivors are particularly susceptible to vaginal atrophy, with up to 62 percent of breast cancer patients reporting severe vaginal dryness in the menopausal period.

Although the majority of women with ovarian cancer are menopausal at the time of diagnosis, approximately one-third are premenopausal. Traditionally, surgical treatment for ovarian cancer involves hysterectomy (removal of the uterus) and bilateral salpingo-oophorectomy (removal of the tubes and ovaries), which causes immediate surgical menopause. This surgery results in abrupt loss of estrogen production by the ovaries, with symptoms that are magnified when compared to symptoms of the natural menopausal transition. Women diagnosed with and treated for ovarian cancer suffer from all the menopausal symptoms listed above, and may be at increased risk due to the abrupt drop in circulating estrogen levels. In addition, the physical changes associated with surgery, including scar tissue formation, the appearance of the skin incision, and fear of bleeding with intercourse may directly affect sexual function and interfere with personal relationships.

Hormone Replacement Therapy

To manage the symptoms of menopause and the increased risk of osteoporosis, many women consider starting HRT. Unfortunately, there is a significant reluctance to begin hormonal therapy after a diagnosis of ovarian cancer, because patients and their medical providers are concerned that taking hormones might stimulate residual cancer or induce a new hormone-dependent disease. This concern is based on experiments with ovarian cancer cell lines (meaning in cultures in the lab, not in humans), which indicated that estrogen promoted cell growth and survival. This has not been shown in human studies.

In several studies exploring the relationship between hormone replacement therapy and survival after a diagnosis of ovarian cancer, no association between HRT and adverse outcome (decreased survival) was shown. Patients who took hormones for menopausal symptoms did not experience more frequent disease recurrence and on average lived as long as their counterparts who did not take hormones (either estrogen or progesterone). These studies are limited because of the small number of patients, although a large randomized trial designed to definitively answer this question is unlikely. Additionally, one study specifically examined patients with estrogen-expressing ovarian cancer cells (removed at the time of surgery), and these women were no more likely to develop recurrence of their cancer in the setting of hormone replacement therapy.

Taking these findings into account, it is our practice to discuss estrogen replacement therapy as a viable option with patients after surgery and treatment for ovarian cancer. The decision to start estrogen therapy is *not* a long-term commitment. At any time, the dose and duration of therapy can be adjusted.

There are various formulations and routes of administration for hormone replacement therapy. Each has its own set of advantages and potential side effects, and the patient and her medical provider should discuss these pros and cons thoroughly. All HRT products require a prescription from your health care practitioner, if he or she believes that estrogen replacement is recommended for you.

Commonly used estrogens are

- conjugated equine estrogen (CEE): Premarin
- micronized estradiol: Estrace
- estropipate (estrogen sulfate): Ogen, Ortho-Est

- ethinyl estradiol: Gynodiol
- estradiol valerate: Delestrogen
- esterified estrogens: Menest

In addition to the oral formulations, low-dose vaginal estrogens are available. These treat primarily the local symptoms of vaginal atrophy, without providing a sufficient systemic dose to address other menopausal symptoms. In the population of women primarily suffering from vaginal atrophy, the vaginal formulation may represent an excellent option. This therapeutic advantage is based on the preponderance of estrogen receptors in the vagina, vulva (external genitalia), labia, and urethra. Additionally, the regimen can be individualized to the patient, with close clinical follow-up.

The following vaginal estrogen formulations are available:

- Estring: 2mg estradiol ring (7.5mcg/day) placed in the upper one-third of the vagina and replaced after 90 days.
- Vagifem: 10mcg tablet placed using the applicator included in the packaging, daily for two weeks to start, with a maintenance dose of one tablet vaginally twice per week.
- Premarin/Estrace: 0.5g to 2g vaginal cream applied intravaginally every day for one to two weeks, then 0.5g twice-weekly maintenance.

The traditional oral and transvaginal routes have more recently been supplemented by transdermal formulations, implants, and nasal estrogen formulations. Of these, the transdermal approach is most commonly used. A steady dose of hormones is supplied by the patch, which is applied to the skin and replaced once or twice each week.

Transdermal estrogen formulations are

- Vivelle Dot: 0.025mg to 0.05mg per day in an estradiol patch applied once or twice per week (doses are available up to 0.1mg per day; we sometimes will give higher doses, such as 0.75mg to 0.1mg per day for our young patients for a short time)
- Climara, Alora, Minivelle, and Menostar (alternate forms of estradiol transdermal)

Alternatives to Hormonal Therapy

For a subset of patients, estrogen therapy may not be an appropriate option, due to existing medical conditions, such as active breast cancer, blood clot, or stroke, or for personal reasons. Additionally, some women may be apprehensive about taking hormonal therapy irrespective of the scientific data, in fear that the hormones may result in side effects or lead to recurrence of their ovarian cancer.

For these women, alternate therapeutic modalities exist. Although less effective than estrogen in ameliorating menopausal symptoms, nonhormonal agents have been documented to be successful. Selective estrogen receptor modulators (SERMs) are a class of drug that helps protect against osteoporosis in postmenopausal women without stimulating estrogen receptors in other tissues. Raloxifene, a commonly used SERM, has the additional benefit of preventing invasive breast cancer and osteoporosis in postmenopausal women. Its drawback, however, is that it does not help with hot flashes, and in some women, it may worsen symptoms.

Phytoestrogens are plant-derived estrogen-like compounds that are taken orally and that act similarly to the estrogen formulations discussed above. Unfortunately, these drugs are 1,000 to 10,000 times less potent than estrogens and are not regulated by the FDA, making quality assurance difficult.

Most commonly, prescriptive alternatives to estrogen-based therapies are used in the treatment of hot flashes and vaginal atrophy. Prescription options include clonidine, venlafaxine (Effexor), and gabapentin. Clonidine, traditionally used to treat high blood pressure, has been shown to reduce hot flashes in postmenopausal women. Unfortunately, despite availability in both oral and patch forms, its long list of associated side effects makes it difficult to use. Effexor is a selective serotonin reuptake inhibitor that is commonly used in the treatment of depression and anxiety. In scientific studies, Effexor, at a dose of 37.5mg per day resulted in a 60 percent reduction in hot flashes. As many cancer survivors commonly deal with depression and anxiety during treatment and while in remission, Effexor is a popular non-estrogen option in the treatment of hot flashes. Gabapentin (Neurontin) is a drug used for the treatment of partial seizures, postherpetic neuralgia, neuropathic pain, and restless leg syndrome. In well-designed studies, oral gabapentin at a dose of 300mg three times per day led to a 50 percent reduction in hot flashes.

Nonhormonal options for the treatment of atrophic vaginitis, or vaginal atrophy, have been less thoroughly studied than those used for hot flashes. One study found that vitamin E and phytoestrogen applied locally as a gel improved symptoms of atrophy. Additionally, oral vitamin D supplementation was found to significantly reduce incidence of vaginal atrophy in women who did not have cancer. Most commonly, women who elect to avoid vaginal estrogens use over-the-counter lubricants and moisturizers, which are water based and available as liquids, gels, or ovules inserted every few days. The moisturizers can be used safely over a long period but must be used regularly for optimal effect. Lubricants, on the other hand, are shorter acting and must be reapplied regularly during intercourse to reduce pain with intercourse (known as *dyspareunia*). Two lubricants commonly used are Replens and Astroglide, with the ultimate decision resting on personal preference, cost, and product availability.

The Decision

Ultimately, as with all interventions and medications, it is important for patients to discuss available options thoroughly with their medical provider. Every woman's situation is composed of a unique set of physical, emotional, and medical needs, and therapy must be tailored to address each one. As mentioned previously, despite the safety of hormone replacement, some women may be apprehensive to take oral estrogen or use a topical formulation, and in those instances nonhormonal alternatives should be explored. Importantly, however, women being treated for ovarian cancer and women in remission should be aware that no strong scientific evidence exists linking oral estrogen with recurrence of ovarian cancer. Conversely, the majority of available data refute the association, indicating that oral estrogen replacement is safe in this setting.

Complementary and Alternative Medicine

As cancer survivorship continues to improve in response to novel therapeutics and improved surgical and supportive care, an increased awareness of managing treatment-related side effects has emerged. Women with ovarian cancer commonly report cancer-related fatigue, nausea, poor sleep, decreased energy, and change in appetite. These side effects in combination with the cancer diagnosis can ultimately result in depression, anxiety, and a sense of loss of control.

Recently, the focus of cancer-based research (drug discovery) has evolved to include patient-reported quality-of-life (QOL) outcomes. This has enabled us, as providers, to understand the intricacies of treatment and to begin to incorporate patient-reported outcomes into ovarian cancer clinical trials. Emerging from this evolution is an understanding that exercise and physical activity, both traditional and in the form of yoga, Pilates, Tai Chi, and dance therapy, can result in improved QOL, which may ultimately prolong survival.

In clinical trials, ovarian cancer patients who reported meeting healthy physical activity guidelines had less cancer-related fatigue, better sleep, and improved psychosocial functioning and overall quality of life. More significant, ovarian cancer patients themselves viewed physical activity as important, with the majority of queried women preferring to start an exercise program within one year of completing treatment, and 31 percent preferring to start during therapy. In a study of 57 patients with ovarian cancer, a six-month exercise intervention was associated with improved aerobic fitness and QOL, as well as a reduction in stress, anxiety, and depression.

In another study, 17 women with newly diagnosed ovarian cancer were recruited to enroll in a walking exercise intervention throughout chemotherapy. The average age of women participating in the study was 60 years, and the majority (88 percent) had Stage III or IV ovarian cancer. On average, the women adhered to more than 80 percent of their intervention sessions and reported improvements in physical function, symptoms, physical well-being, and ovarian cancer–specific quality of life. Additionally, 76 percent of the women enrolled in the study completed all assigned chemotherapy treatment, supporting earlier research indicating that physical activity may be associated with an improved ability to complete treatment.

When looking at studies of all cancer patients (not only those with ovarian cancer)—a total of 56 trials with more than 4,800 participants—exercise (walking, cycling, resistance or strength training) resulted in improved quality of life and social functioning and decreased fatigue. Importantly, as with all scientific findings, these results need to be interpreted with caution, as the exercise programs were variable across studies, and how quality of life was measured varied. Nonetheless, given the relatively low risk of a moderate exercise program, and the possible benefits, we encourage women with ovarian cancer to participate in physical activity, appropriate to their ability and level of health. In our practice, physical activity and health is promoted strongly throughout therapy and during surveillance.

Sleep-Wake Disturbances

Many women with ovarian cancer report significant sleep-wake disturbances. When taking a comprehensive medical history, the physician will try to determine whether the sleep disturbance was present before diagnosis or only began after surgery and chemotherapy. The physician will also want to know whether the patient has difficulty falling asleep or staying asleep, with an inability to return to sleep. Also important is whether the patient feels rested after awakening for the day. Women who have frequent night sweats from menopause may awaken several times during the night, with or without returning to sleep, and remain tired during daytime hours. Naps during the day, which can interfere with falling asleep at scheduled night hours, may be a cause of sleep disturbances.

Fatigue is a common result of interrupted sleep for many people, even those without a cancer diagnosis. Sorting out all the contributing factors of fatigue are the first steps in helping patients improve their energy. Patients who report fatigue need to be assessed for medical reasons, such as anemia from chemotherapy, thyroid imbalance, pain, depression, sleep apnea, and stimulant medications. Fatigue can be a result of a sleep disorder or a sleep schedule interruption.

Because persistent fatigue will interfere with self-management of daily living activities and with achieving a positive frame of mind, the health care team and the patient need to discuss, and address, sleep problems and fatigue. In discussing sleep problems, many patients will identify it as insomnia. Once questions about the onset of the problems are answered, including whether the problems are acute (less than a month) or chronic (one month or longer), the patient may be asked to keep a sleep diary in which she records her sleep and wake hours to help identify a pattern to her sleep disturbances. Another way for patients to identify an interrupted pattern of sleep is to use a sleep-recording device in the form of a wristband. Such devices monitor fitness goals and sleep patterns and are synced with a personal computer or smartphone. Some patients have insomnia due to worry and anxiety about their cancer, financial burdens, or other life stressors. If anxiety is a contributing factor, stress reduction may be the most useful intervention, whether on your own or with a qualified therapist. It may take time and commitment to achieve a comfortable level of stress.

There is limited research on the effectiveness of complementary therapies for the improvement of sleep disorders related to stress and anxiety. Some suggested interventions that may be helpful include mindfulness-based stress reduction, guided imagery, music therapy, and muscle relaxation. Some women may benefit from working with a therapist who does cognitive-behavioral therapy to treat anxiety (ask your physician about a referral).

Sleep-wake disturbances due to hot flashes can be burdensome for patients, especially if they require changing clothes or bedsheets due to excessive sweating during the night. Your health care practitioner may prescribe a short-term course of estrogen replacement if the hot flashes are frequent and disruptive to sleep, and if there are no contraindications within your specific health history (as described above). Other interventions include having a fan by the bedside and using a cooling pillow or cooling blanket, which can be purchased at specialty stores or from online stores. Melatonin (N-acetyl-5-methoxytryptamine), a naturally occurring hormone categorized as a dietary supplement by the FDA, is involved in regulating circadian rhythms and may be a useful sleep aid. Melatonin can be obtained over the counter; however, the effects of long-term supplementation have not been fully studied.

Prescription sleeping pills are often used for sleep-wake disturbances. This approach may be effective for many patients, even though it fails to identify or address the cause of the sleep disturbance. In some situations, patients require higher doses of sleep medications because their body develops a tolerance to, or becomes used to, the prescribed medication dose. It is important to communicate with your health care team if your prescribed dose of medication is no longer effective. Only under the management of your health care provider is it ever recommended for patients to increase the dose of sleeping pills. Patients should not add other agents such as benzodiazepines or herbal supplements to improve sleep without first discussing it with their health care team. Interventions may require a combination of treatment approaches, including stress reduction and medication support, to find the effective modality to improve sleep-wake disturbances and thereby improve emotional and physical health.

Cognitive or Memory Changes

Many patients report cognitive impairment during treatment or after completion of chemotherapy. Affectionately called "chemobrain" by patients, this real phenomenon creates forgetfulness and difficulty in multitasking, retrieving words, and comprehension. It can alter a patient's decision making and cognitive performance at home or at work. Most patients report noticeable memory changes or mild cognitive impairment after chemotherapy, which can linger for two, three, even four years after chemotherapy. Changes can be subtle, and friends and family may not even notice any difference, but patients find it distressing. Some patients express concern that they fear a brain tumor or mental illness.

Most of the research on chemotherapy-induced cognitive changes has been conducted on women with breast cancer, although there are studies of patients with other types of cancer, including ovarian cancer. Cognitive change measurements can be validated with neurocognitive tests and complex imaging modalities. Even though routine cognitive testing is not performed except under the protocol of a clinical trial, or with a neurologist or neuropsychologist specialist, patients can be reassured that chemo-brain is real and that their memory changes will improve over time.

Factors that may be associated with chemotherapy-related cognitive changes include older age, anxiety, depression, aggressive chemotherapy regimens, disease site and stage, and biochemical and medical conditions. It can be difficult to differentiate whether compounding factors are contributing to or are the cause of the memory changes. For example, pain medications or steroids can cause short-term behavior and cognitive changes. Fatigue and inadequate sleep can contribute to forgetfulness and memory changes, as can inadequate nutrition and hydration. Increased age is associated with a greater decline in memory, unrelated to a cancer diagnosis and treatment. Yet younger patients, especially premenopausal women who have surgically induced menopause followed by chemotherapy, may have an increased perception of cognitive change, and therefore an additional effect on quality of life.

Many patients have reported the typical scenario of walking into a room and forgetting what they wanted from the room in the first place. This happens to all people, even without a cancer diagnosis, but is reported more commonly by women who have undergone chemotherapy for ovarian or breast cancer. Other examples include stopping midsentence in a conversation and forgetting the primary train of thought. The inability to remember words when conversing is also a common phenomenon. Women also describe a fogginess and the inability to stay focused on a project, even though they could easily focus prior to receiving chemotherapy. Although there is no rapid or definite remedy for chemo-brain, organizational strategies such as keeping lists, calendars, and alerts and reminders on electronic devices; playing brain-stimulating games such as crossword puzzles and Scrabble; or engaging in a hobby may be beneficial. Practicing simple math such as balancing a checkbook without a calculator is another example of a stimulating brain activity. If symptoms persist or become sufficiently distressful for a patient, a referral to a neuropsychologist, often at a research-focused academic hospital, can facilitate cognitive testing and development of cognitive and coping skills.

There are no medications approved for chemo-brain, but some medications, such as methylphenidate (Ritalin) for attention deficit disorder or modafinal (Provigil) for narcolepsy, have been reported to help individuals with cognitive changes. Other tips include keeping a diary of when you notice changes, to help identify how often cognitive changes occur and whether there is an identifiable pattern (such as when you are stressed, multitasking, or in a rush). This diary can then be shared with your health care team to determine if other things can be done. Poly-pharmacy (taking multiple medications while on treatment) can affect cognitive function. Bring a list of all your medications, including supplements, to your physician appointment. Before seeing your practitioner, make a list of questions and, if possible, bring a friend or family member to appointments. Write down the answers to your questions or ask your practitioner if you can audio-record the visit. If you notice changes in memory or cognitive function, you should always share this information with your health care team. Learning to adapt and cope with memory changes can be frustrating, but with time it will become easier.

Mind-Body Wellness

The term *mind-body therapy* is somewhat ambiguous but generally refers to a group of treatments that work to treat both the *psyche* (mind) and the *soma* (body). Many of these modalities fall under the category of complementary and alternative therapies, which are used by up to one-third of cancer patients. For care to be comprehensive, providers and patients need to get comfortable about discussing these nontraditional interventions and to open a dialogue about how useful they might be.

Data regarding mind-body techniques are limited. Here we briefly review those modalities with data indicating usefulness in cancer survivors.

Hypnosis, initially introduced by Franz Anton Mesmer two hundred years ago, has been shown to benefit cancer patients, improving cancer-related pain and relieving chemotherapy-induced nausea and vomiting. It is hypothesized that the effects of hypnosis are mediated through muscle relaxation, perceptual alterations, and cognitive distraction.

A more comprehensive approach is employed in an intervention known as mindfulness-based stress reduction (MBSR). This intervention incorporates meditation, yoga, and stress reduction. In clinical trials, MBSR resulted in improvement in mood disturbance and in decreased stress. Perhaps more important, patients enrolled in the stress reduction program exhibited a transition in their immune cell profile and a decreased depressive profile. The implications of an immune transition may be underappreciated, as we are only now beginning to discover the pivotal role immune function may play in the treatment of advanced-stage ovarian cancer.

Tai Chi, a series of postures and movements along with controlled breathing, has also been investigated in patients with a cancer diagnosis. Despite a lack of controlled clinical trials, two studies in breast cancer survivors have associated Tai Chi with improvement in psychological and physiological symptoms. The list of other potential interventions targeting mind-body wellness includes art therapy, massage, acupuncture, and neuro-emotional techniques. As Western medicine continues to explore these therapeutic alternatives, it will be important to study the implications of such interventions on both quality of life and survival.

Theory of Inner Strength

Fortunately, cancer survival rates are increasing, but not all cancer survivors are without burdens. It is believed that patients will go through many stages, such as anguish and fear, as they search for meaning and process the diagnosis of cancer. Health care practitioners are committed not only to their patients' survival outcomes, but also to maintaining quality of life and promoting a desire to keep living. Defining quality of life is personal, and we are discovering that patients who report a high QOL are those who have or develop a positive concept of rebuilding one's self after going through a challenging life event such as cancer. The support system from relationships with family and friends, a health care team, as well as spiritual beliefs can help a cancer survivor develop her inner strength. A relationship with self is also part of that support system: the ability to love yourself and not blame yourself for things that you wish you could have done differently. The next stage is engaging in possibilities, realizing that you will set your mind to fighting through treatment, achieving a positive outlook, and finding your new normal. It will be a transition, something that will take time. As mentioned in other chapters, psychological and emotional changes are likely to occur at some point during treatment, and possibly at completion of treatment. The more time that passes from initial diagnosis, the less anxious you will feel, with a decline in feelings of distress and depression. Self-management and independence are health outcome goals, but support from others, including communication with your health care team, is part of working toward inner strength.

Spirituality serves as a source of comfort for many people. The belief in a higher power, or in destiny (all things happen for a reason), is unique to an individual's search for and understanding of meaning and purpose. Spirituality and religion may mean different things to different people. Religion is often a set of beliefs within an organized group, while spirituality is usually more ambiguous and represents an individual's personal beliefs. You do not need to belong to a religion or group to be spiritual.

Spirituality can provide hope and a sense of control in coping with a cancer diagnosis. Spiritual distress can hinder coping if an individual believes she has cancer because God is punishing her for not living life in a different way. Some patients believe they did something wrong in their life that made God give them cancer. The health care team supports the personal beliefs of the patient, regardless of the faith base of the practitioner. If you want to add spiritual guidance to your life, or have unresolved questions, your health care team can make referrals to clergy in the cancer center or hospital, or refer you to spiritual mentors closer to your home. Modalities such as meditation, guided imagery, yoga, and other calming influences can help support spiritual growth.

Conclusion

Increasingly, the treatment of women with ovarian cancer has moved well beyond the traditional focus on surgery followed by selecting and administering drugs (chemotherapy). Patient quality of life during treatment and in the survivorship phase is becoming increasingly important. We believe women should be helped to feel empowered and to have an understanding of their options, as they relate to the treatment of menopausal symptoms, the effects of exercise on quality of life, and overall mind-body wellness.

CHAPTER 9

Integrative Medicine for Ovarian Cancer

Diljeet K. Singh, MD, DrPH, and Mario Javier Pineda, MD, PhD

In spite of the progress we have made in the treatment of ovarian cancer, living with this diagnosis remains a challenge. As a survivor, you are naturally exploring all the options you have to improve your cancer outcomes and to maximize your quality of life. In this chapter we hope to give you guidance as you explore interventions and modalities that might be outside the traditional realm of gynecologic oncology.

Definitions

The National Institutes of Health National Center for Complementary and Integrative Health defines *complementary medicine* as "a group of diverse medical and health care systems, practices, and products that are not generally considered part of conventional medicine" but that are practiced in conjunction with conventional care. *Alternative therapies,* by contrast, are typically promoted as a substitute for mainstream care; by definition, they have not been scientifically proved, often have no scientific foundation, and sometimes have even been disproved. The concept of integrative medicine has evolved to describe the combination of conventional medicine with complementary medical practices for which there is evidence of safety and effectiveness.

The Consortium of Academic Health Centers for Integrative Medicine defines integrative medicine as "the practice of medicine that reaffirms the importance of the relationship between practitioner and patient, focuses on the whole person, is informed by evidence, and makes use of all appropriate therapeutic approaches, health care professionals, and disciplines to achieve optimal health and healing." Integrative oncology focuses on the complex health of people with cancer and proposes an array of approaches to accompany the conventional therapies. We encourage you to think of integrative oncology as both a science and a philosophy, focused on your well-being by proposing multiple approaches to be used along with conventional therapies to improve health.

In this chapter we cover many (though not all) of the numerous approaches of integrative medicine. In table 9.1 we group the different approaches into six commonly used categories and give examples of each.

Can Improving Lifestyle Improve Cancer Outcomes?

Many people with cancer wonder whether lifestyle makes any difference, or whether "the damage has already been done." The earliest research on diet and exercise was focused on cancer prevention; more recent work, however, focused on cancer survivors, and this work also showed benefits from improvements in lifestyle, with better cancer-related outcomes and enhanced quality of life (figure 9.1). A healthy and balanced diet, regular exercise, stress management, social support, regular sleep, and avoidance of tobacco have all shown benefit. The most data come from studying people who have more common cancers like breast and prostate cancers, but these findings are relevant to ovarian cancer survivors because of the inherent similarities between cancers in general and cancers that seem to be influenced by sex hormones.

One project evaluating men who have early prostate cancer showed that the combination of a low-fat, plant-based diet; regu-

TABLE 9.1 *Six Common Categories of Integrative Medicine*

Categories of Approaches	Examples
Diet and lifestyle modifications	Mediterranean diet, anti-inflammatory diet, exercise regimens
Natural products and supplements	Herbs, botanicals, vitamins, minerals, antioxidants
Mind-body interventions	Yoga, mindfulness meditation-based stress reduction, music therapy, hypnosis, meditation, prayer, guided imagery, Qigong/Tai Chi Chuan
Energy medicine	Reiki, therapeutic touch
Manual medicine	Massage, chiropractic, reflexology
Alternative medical systems	Naturopathy, homeopathy, traditional Chinese medicine and acupuncture, Ayurvedic medicine

lar aerobic exercise; stress management techniques; and support group involvement decreased the likelihood of needing to go on to additional cancer treatment, such as surgery, radiation, or anti-testosterone treatment. The Women's Healthy Eating and Living Study evaluated women with early-stage breast cancer and showed

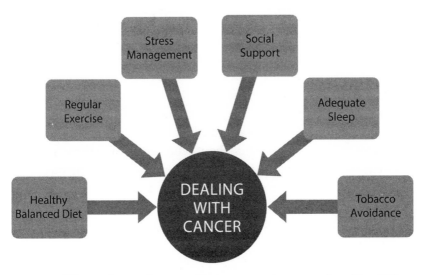

FIGURE 9.1 Lifestyle factors that can affect cancer outcomes and quality of life.

that a combination of eating five or more fruits and vegetables per day and doing physical activity equivalent to walking 30 minutes per day, six days per week, was associated with significantly better survival. A study of physical activity in ovarian cancer patients showed that as activity increased, fatigue, peripheral neuropathy, mood disturbance, and sleep disturbance all decreased. In addition, the most active women reported more happiness and better sleep quality. All this evidence supports the idea that even after a cancer develops, how we live matters.

What Is Right for You? Considering Risks and Benefits

As a cancer survivor, you may be targeted by unethical practitioners who are focused more on making money than on treating cancer, so you need to approach practitioners and interventions with caution. In addition, some practitioners may truly believe in the efficacy of an approach that has little research behind it or that has not been used in ovarian cancer survivors. Miracle cures and instant fixes are often disappointing wastes of time and money and sometimes of well-being.

Choosing a Provider

Go about choosing an integrative health care provider in the same way you would approach choosing a doctor (see tables 9.2 and 9.3). Consider getting referrals from your oncologist or hospital or cancer center, or contact officially recognized professional or government organizations to get the names of certified practitioners. When you meet with practitioners, be sure to ask them about their training and licensure. Talk to practitioners about what types of approaches they practice; what the risks, side effects, and possible benefits might be; and whether they have previously taken care of women with ovarian cancer. Make sure practitioners are willing to work with your team and be sure they understand what your goals are in seeking their assistance.

TABLE 9.2   *Questions to Ask Integrative Providers*

What types of modalities do you use?
What are your training and qualifications?
Do you see other patients with my type of cancer?
Will you work with my doctor?
How can this help me?
Do you know of studies that prove it helps?
What are the risks and side effects?
Can this interfere with my cancer treatment?
Will my insurance cover the treatment?
What will it cost?
Do you have information that I can read about it?
Are there any reasons I should not use it?

TABLE 9.3   *Questions to Ask Yourself about Integrative Providers and Their Approaches*

Do I feel comfortable with this person?
Do I like how the office looks and feels?
Do I like the staff?
Does this person support standard cancer treatments?
What are my goals in taking on this approach?
Do I understand the risks?

The Best Available Data for You

One of the struggles in obtaining health care is getting good information about the potential benefits and risks of a given intervention. Getting the data is especially difficult when it comes to integrative medicine. Data from well-conducted studies are limited, for several reasons. Until recently, much of integrative medicine was considered "fringe" or "quackery," certainly outside the realm of science, so studies of this work were not undertaken. In 1992 the National Institutes of Health finally developed a consistent source of guidance and funding for research and training in integrative medicine, and at this time research was initiated.

Another factor is that the Food and Drug Administration regulates dietary supplements as foods, not drugs, so it does not analyze the content or ingredients of supplements. This means that supplements may not be consistent in quality or ingredients. For example, a supplement may not contain the same amount of the herb or other ingredient, resulting in significant variability from bottle to bottle and brand to brand. This status also means that pharmaceutical companies cannot get patents on supplements, so they have limited incentive for research. Furthermore, natural sources are hard to study, because plants have many parts, including seeds, roots, stems, leaves, and flowers, all of which may have important and differing properties.

Finally, alternative health systems, such as Ayurvedic medicine and traditional Chinese medicine, have different concepts of health and well-being and may approach both diagnosis and treatment differently from how they are approached in allopathic medicine (a term for conventional Western medicine). For example, an acupuncturist may be focusing on balancing "chi," while the referring oncologist may believe he or she is sending a patient to get help with managing chemotherapy-related nausea. These differing perspectives can potentially serve you as an individual; however, they can make research difficult.

Just as you discuss with your oncologist the risks and benefits of chemotherapy or surgery, you should look at these aspects of any other treatments you consider and put them in the context of your current health and goals (figure 9.2). For example, a protein-restrictive diet that may otherwise be safe can hinder healing after a major surgical procedure. Clearly, a great deal of additional research must be conducted to fully evaluate integrative approaches. However, working with your health care team, including physician, pharmacists, and nurses, you can take a "best available data for me" approach.

What to Be Aware of When Looking at Herbs and Supplements

As mentioned above, the quality of herbal preparations is not well governed, and contamination of preparations has been reported. Reported cases of complications with herb use are quite rare, however, and safe, effective products can be identified with trained guidance. You should let your oncologist know what supplements you are considering or already taking, because many herbs may potentially cause

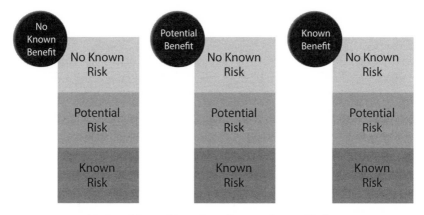

FIGURE 9.2 Considering risks and benefits of integrative medical treatments.

allergic reactions and significantly interact with over-the-counter and prescription drugs. Often a pharmacist on the team can help figure out what side effects and drug interactions might occur, what is safe, and what should be avoided.

We know that some supplements can increase or decrease the effectiveness of other medications by changing how the body handles them. Herbs such as kava and valerian can heighten the sedative effect of anesthetics. St. John's wort influences the liver to break down many drugs faster, including warfarin, irinotecan, cyclosporine, oral contraceptives, digitalis, midazolam, lidocaine, and calcium channel blockers. Echinacea, goldenseal, and licorice may slow the breakdown of these same medications so that they will have longer-lasting, possibly stronger effects. Chondroitin, evening primrose, gingko biloba, garlic, ginseng, ginger, green tea concentrated pills, fish and flaxseed oils, vitamin E, dong quai, and feverfew can all affect our ability to clot, which can lead to a risk of bleeding. Supplements that can influence our cardiovascular system include ephedra and pharmacological doses of garlic.

Several studies suggest that omega-3 fatty acids (contained in fish oil), which is a commonly taken supplement, have anti-inflammatory properties, may prevent tumor growth, and may reduce chemotherapy side effects. However, there are also small studies indicating that fish oil in the doses found in pills may interfere with chemotherapy.

Getting omega-3 fatty acids by eating olive oil and oily fish, such as sardines and salmon, at least three times a week is likely the safest thing to do while on active chemotherapy. When taken with a physician's recommendation, fish oil supplements are probably safe and may have significant potential for benefit. Ultimately, you and your team need to use your best judgment regarding what herbs and supplements are reasonable for you. Whole foods remain the best way to get your nutrients and can provide safe, healthy, and often delicious sources of nutrients that can support your well-being and improve your cancer outcomes.

What to Think about When Considering Dietary Approaches

How and what we eat every day plays a role in our health and our cancer risk. In addition, several studies have shown that food choices we make after cancer is diagnosed are also important. Separating the role of whole foods eaten as part of a general diet and supplements taken in addition to whole foods is difficult in research and in practice, which means that much of the information we have is imperfect. Several diets have gained considerable popularity among people diagnosed with cancer; reviewing them in detail is outside the scope of this chapter. Ovarian cancer survivors should beware of any diet that excludes major nutrients. During and after cancer treatment, your focus should be on making sure you choose whole foods that are not processed or refined and that have a variety of different colors and tastes so that you get the broadest range of nutrients possible. Do not spend a lot of time and worry on the occasional (once a week at most) "unhealthy" food you eat.

In addition, having cancer and being treated for it can put you at risk for nutritional deficiencies. For example, if a significant portion of the small intestine (*terminal ileum*) is removed, absorption of vitamin B_{12} may be decreased. Consulting a dietitian or nutritional specialist can be beneficial in identifying areas of risk and promoting optimal health.

How the Research Gets Done: The Example of the Mediterranean Diet

The earliest research on diet and cancer focused on regions known for having lower cancer rates and evaluated the diet of the people who lived there. Some of the interesting data we have on the Mediterranean diet, an excellent diet choice for ovarian cancer survivors, come from this work. Diets of the people living around the Mediterranean Sea have common features, which include high consumption of omega-3 fatty acids (in the form of olive oil, fish, and nuts), protein predominantly from plant and fish sources, high consumption of fruits and vegetables, low consumption of red meat, low to moderate dairy consumption, and moderate regular consumption of red wine. These studies found that the people living in these areas lived longer and had less chance of having heart disease, cancer, or strokes than people who did not live in this area of the world. The trouble with understanding what this means is that other things also affect all the people in the area—such as the air, weather, water, and sun exposure—so it may be difficult to give all the credit for good outcomes to what people eat.

The next steps in this research were to determine what components of the diet seemed to matter most and whether being more adherent to the diet increased its benefits. This kind of dietary research is tricky for various reasons. Researchers get dietary information from people who either have to recall what they ate in the past or have to keep track of what they are eating now using diet diaries. As anyone who has tried to keep track of calories knows, there is room for error in everything from judging serving size to remembering everything you ate, and it is all influenced by an element of wishful thinking. When this next step of evaluation was done on the Mediterranean diet, scientists found that the people who adhered to the diet most faithfully had significantly lower chances of developing cancer and of dying from it. Researchers examined the relationship between the gynecologic cancers and specific components of the Mediterranean diet and found a significantly decreased risk for endometrial and ovarian cancers with higher vegetable intake. The highest consumption level of whole grains was also associated with a decreased risk for endometrial and ovarian cancers. The risk for ovarian cancer was lower in women who had a higher intake of omega-3 fatty acids. Finally, women who had a higher red meat intake had a higher chance of developing endometrial and ovarian cancers.

Dietary researchers also try to figure out the biology behind the benefits, and this is the work that can lead to a focus on supplements rather than whole foods. With the Mediterranean diet, scientists think that the health benefits are based on several bioactive compounds (compounds that have an effect on a living organism, tissue, or cell but that are not essential for survival) and their interactions, including the omega-3 fats in olive oil, fish, and nuts; the high fiber content of fruits, vegetables, and whole grains; and the phytonutrients and antioxidants in many components of the diet. Of note, the benefit of red wine may be related to the resveratrol that comes from grapes, and in women the benefit is likely outweighed by the breast cancer–related risk of regular alcohol intake. Even just a daily glass of wine has been shown to increase the risk of breast cancer in women.

Once specific foods are found to be important, studies in different populations are examined to see whether the same results are found in these different settings. In one study of more than 300 women with ovarian cancer, longer survival was seen in those who had the best intake of fruits and vegetables. Researchers found that yellow and cruciferous vegetables (broccoli, cauliflower, kale, cabbage, bok choy, arugula) seemed to be important. Other work has shown that glucosinolates, crambene, indole-3-carbinol, and isothiocyanates (compounds contained in cruciferous vegetables) decrease the risk of developing cancer and likely account, in part, for the benefits of these vegetables. A second study of more than 600 women with epithelial ovarian cancer who were followed for five years confirmed that women with higher intake of vegetables and especially cruciferous vegetables had better survival. Bringing together multiple studies, researchers showed that a low intake of processed meats (such as bacon and other nitrate-preserved meats) and a higher consumption of fish and poultry could decrease a woman's chance of getting ovarian cancer. A study in New York showed that the following dietary components seemed to decrease a woman's chance of getting ovarian cancer: fiber, vegetables, poultry, beta-carotene (a vitamin A precursor found in oranges and yellow fruits and vegetables), stigmasterol (a plant fat in seeds, nuts, and legumes), and *lignans* (a compound with weak estrogenic properties found in seeds, whole grains, legumes, fruits, and vegetables). Women who had a higher kaempferol intake (a plant phytonutrient found in tea, broccoli, grapefruit, cabbage, kale, beans, endives, leeks, tomatoes, strawberries, grapes, brussels sprouts, and apples) had less chance of getting ovarian cancer, as did women who had a higher luteonlin content in their diets (a plant phytonutrient found in celery, broccoli, green peppers, parsley, thyme, chamomile, carrots, olive oil, peppermint, rosemary, oranges, and oregano). Although these studies provide important clues in understanding cancer and cancer prevention, ultimately, whole foods have the best chance of improving health by creating the most effective combinations of phytonutrients.

Are Soy and Other Phytoestrogens Safe?

The research on soy followed a similar path as the studies on the Mediterranean diet, starting with results from population studies looking at cancer prevention and then progressing to following cancer survivors, all while laboratory scientists studied the potentially active parts of the plant. Studies of populations with high whole soy intake showed decreased risk of cancers that are influenced by the female hormones estrogen and progesterone, such as breast cancer, endometrial cancer, and ovarian cancer. A large study that compared the lowest soy intake group to the highest soy intake group showed a 39 percent decrease in the risk of all hormone-related cancers, a 30 percent decrease in the risk of endometrial cancer, and a 48 percent decrease for ovarian cancer in the highest soy intake group.

The active ingredients in soy are thought to be *phytoestrogens*, which are naturally occurring plant substances with chemical structures similar to estrogen. They consist mainly of *isoflavones* (high concentrations in soy beans and other legumes) and lignans (in fruits, vegetables, grains, seeds, and legumes). Isoflavones are weak estrogens compared to estradiol, the more potent ovarian estrogen. The high soy intake and low rates of breast cancer in Asian populations led to the idea that the isoflavones in soy might replace estradiol on cells, causing a functional lower estrogen effect. As we learned about isoflavones, practitioners became concerned that soy intake could be harmful in women with hormonally related cancers who were menopausal and no longer had functioning ovaries; in these women even weak estrogens might be strong enough to stimulate the cancer. So studies were undertaken in women already diagnosed with cancer, and these studies showed that soy was safe and potentially beneficial in women with estrogen-responsive breast cancer. We have not yet done these studies in women who survived ovarian cancer. Until more research is completed, avoid processed soy and soy supplements and pills. The evidence suggests, however, that whole soy products (tofu, tempeh, edamame, soy milk) and phytoestrogens from other whole food sources are at least safe and potentially beneficial in women with hormonally mediated cancers. Many women are unable to convert isoflavones in soy to their bioactive forms, so some researchers encourage fermented soy products, miso and tempeh, which seem to be more bioavailable.

Whole Foods versus Supplements: The Lessons from Vitamins

Considering how important good nutrition is for cancer survivors, adding various vitamins to your daily regimen may seem like the right thing to do; however, research is adding up to indicate that the benefits might be limited and that there may be harms as well. Our national fascination with the multivitamin started when initial reports showed decreased rates of cancer in populations and individuals who had a high intake of whole yellow and orange vegetables and fruits. Laboratory work showed that beta-carotene and its synthetic derivatives in the vitamin A family play a role in guiding cells along pathways of growth and development, so biologically, beta-carotene was thought to be the active cancer-preventive ingredient.

Two large research trials were undertaken using forms of beta-carotene (β-carotene and synthetic vitamin A in the form of retinyl palmitate) as well as vitamin E (dl-α-tocopheryl acetate), and to the researchers' surprise, they found increases in the risk of lung cancer in the study populations that consisted of men and women who were smokers or who were exposed to asbestos. The reasons for this unexpected harm are not clear, though concerns over the doses and the forms of the vitamins have been raised. In addition, the combination of micronutrients in whole foods is likely important to achieving benefits without increasing risk. As described above, beta-carotene and all the forms of vitamin A regulate cell growth and differentiation, so they may affect precancerous or dormant cancer cells. These pathways may explain why their use increased the risk of lung cancer in smokers and could be relevant to ovarian cancer survivors. Based upon the data we have, it is unclear how beta-carotene supplementation would affect an ovarian cancer survivor, regardless of whether she smokes. In 2014, the U.S. Preventive Services Task Force issued recommendations against the use of beta-carotene and vitamin E supplementation (table 9.4). Intake of antioxidants through diets rich in vegetables and fruits is safe and encouraged.

Should You Use Supplemental Antioxidants during Treatment?

Substantial controversy exists over the safety of taking supplemental antioxidants during chemotherapy and radiation. Some practitioners believe that antioxidant supplements are useful with chemotherapy because they improve the effectiveness of the therapy and alleviate toxic side effects, allowing people to get the full course of treatment and at the highest doses. Others have raised the concern

TABLE 9.4   *Vitamin-Related Recommendations from the U.S. Preventive Services Task Force, 2014*

The Task Force concludes that the current evidence is insufficient to assess the balance of benefits and harms of the use of multivitamins for the prevention of cardiovascular disease or cancer.

The Task Force concludes that the current evidence is insufficient to assess the balance of benefits and harms of the use of single- or paired-nutrient supplements (with the exception of beta-carotene and vitamin E) for the prevention of cardiovascular disease or cancer.

The Task Force recommends against the use of beta-carotene or vitamin E supplements for the prevention of cardiovascular disease or cancer. Beta-carotene supplements may increase the chance of getting lung cancer for people who are already at risk of lung cancer, such as smokers.

that antioxidants may decrease the effectiveness of chemotherapy by limiting the damage that chemotherapy can do to cancer cells. This concern that antioxidants will decrease the effectiveness of chemotherapy has not been seen in the studies examining this question. In the majority of studies, patients receiving antioxidants during chemotherapy did not suffer differences in cancer outcome and had fewer side effects.

Evidence for harm with supplements during radiation therapy has been found. In a study examining 540 patients with early head and neck cancer, researchers found that among smokers, antioxidant supplementation using synthetic beta-carotene and vitamin E or vitamin E alone during radiation therapy was associated with significant increases in the chances of cancer recurrence, dying from the cancer, or dying from any cause. What this information means for you as an ovarian cancer survivor is not clear and is ultimately a decision for you, your doctor, and your nutritional consultants to make after weighing the risks and benefits.

Are There "Super Foods"? Food Components and Natural Products as Supplements

As people start thinking about what to eat, they often get focused on "super foods" and the supplements derived from them, especially on the research hinting that some individual dietary components may be important. There is evidence that several foods are important in preventing and possibly in treating the hormonally related cancers (breast, endometrial, ovarian), but most of the information is derived from breast cancer research, not ovarian cancer. See table 9.5 for a summary of commonly used and emerging supplements. It is important to note that for most of these supplements, the data are limited regarding use in ovarian cancer survivors.

What Does Inflammation Have to Do with Cancer?

The term *inflammation* covers a wide range of healthy and unhealthy processes that happen in the body; there is still a great deal of

TABLE 9.5 *Commonly Used Energy Supplements*

	Evidence in Ovarian Cancer	Overview of the Data	Recommendation
Selenium Mineral	Limited	In a very small study, selenium supplementation increased white blood cell counts and appetite and decreased hair loss, abdominal pain, and weakness.	Make sure your diet includes foods rich in selenium, such as Brazil nuts, sunflower seeds, fish (tuna, halibut, sardines, flounder, salmon), shellfish (oysters, mussels, shrimp, clams, scallops), poultry (chicken, turkey), eggs, mushrooms (button, crimini, shiitake), grains (wheat germ, barley, brown rice, oats), and onions.
Curcumin A component of turmeric	Limited	Curcumin concentrates in the gastrointestinal tract, and most studies showing benefit have been in prevention of colonic polyps and colon cancer or treatment of advanced pancreatic cancer.	Oral curcumin is well tolerated, and liberal use of it in the diet in the form of the spice turmeric (which is used in curry powder) is certainly reasonable.

continued

TABLE 9.5 *continued*

	Evidence in Ovarian Cancer	Overview of the Data	Recommendation
Huang qi (*Astragalus membranaceus*)			
A traditional Chinese herbal medicine long used in that tradition for immune support	None	In lung cancer survivors on platinum-based chemotherapy, there were fewer chemotherapy side effects as well as improvements in survival, cancer outcome, general well-being, and ability to perform activities of daily life. Patients with colon cancer had decreased nausea and vomiting and fewer episodes of low white blood cell counts.	Further study is needed before we can make strong recommendations for the use of these supplements. Be sure to discuss use with your oncologist and your pharmacist before taking.
Green tea			
	Adequate	In 2 large studies, habitual green tea intake reduced the risk of ovarian cancer with greater benefits at higher levels of intake. A study of 200 women with epithelial ovarian cancer demonstrated that consistent green tea consumption led to an improvement in cancer outcome that increased with higher intake.	Numerous studies have shown that green tea as a drink (not in pill form) may have potential in preventing and treating cancer.

TABLE 9.5 *continued*

	Evidence in Ovarian Cancer	Overview of the Data	Recommendation
Vitamin D			
	Limited	The research on vitamin D and cancer comes mostly from studies of sun exposure, geography, and blood studies, not from people who were given vitamin D and then followed over time.	All the evidence suggests that having low vitamin D is a concern, but there is no evidence that having *above* normal levels of vitamin D is preventive or improves ovarian cancer survival. Ovarian cancer survivors should have their blood levels checked and, if they are not in the normal range, get adequate supplementation with follow-up blood work as needed.
American ginseng (*Panax quinquefolius*)			
An herb with a long history of use in traditional Chinese medicine to boost energy	Limited	A clinical trial was conducted comparing 2,000mg daily to a placebo in 340 people with various cancers (60% had breast cancer). After 8 weeks of use, the people on ginseng had a 20-point improvement on a 100-point fatigue scale and reported a significant decrease in feelings of being "pooped," "worn out," or "sluggish."	Although no complications were noted in the study, all herb use should be discussed with your physician.

research to be done in this arena. Ovarian cancer survivors should not assume that diets and supplements labeled as "anti-inflammatory" are going to be universally beneficial to them. That said, researchers have found that chronic systemic inflammation contributes to the risk of cancer, providing an environment that allows cancer cells to survive locally, to grow into neighboring areas (a process known as invasion), and to metastasize. Inflammation itself is a healthy part of responding to infection and injury. However, two main factors in modern life, diet and stress, have increased the biological processes and chemicals that lead to inflammation in situations that do not benefit from these changes.

How Diet Contributes to Inflammation

Many aspects of the modern diet contribute to inflammation, cancer risk, and cancer outcomes, including the kinds of carbohydrates, fats, and proteins we eat. Glycemic index measures how quickly and by how much a food raises blood glucose levels; when the blood glucose level rises, it leads the body to produce insulin, a process called a *chemical cascade*. Insulin has numerous stimulating effects directly on cells, as well as on other chemical cascades. Bread, white potatoes, crackers, chips, pastries, sweetened drinks, refined and processed foods, fast foods, and products made with high-fructose corn syrup all have high glycemic indexes. Researchers have shown that diets with high glycemic indexes increase the risk of getting ovarian cancer as well as other cancers. Biologically, numerous pathways are thought to contribute to this risk, including the stimulating effects on cell growth of high insulin levels and the related factors that insulin triggers. This insulin/insulin-related factor pathway may also be one of the reasons that being overweight or obese increases the chance of getting ovarian cancer.

Omega-3 fatty acids are the building blocks of the biochemicals that turn off inflammation, and omega-6 fatty acids are the building blocks of the biochemicals that support the inflammatory process. As we have evolved in our ability to cultivate food, the balance of omega-3 to omega-6 fatty acids in our diet has shifted: from a 1 to 1 balance when we were hunter-gatherers to a 1 to 8 ratio in the 1930s and now to a 1 to 25 ratio. This imbalance means our diet is feeding the pro-inflammatory process and starving the anti-inflammatory pathways. Omega-6 fatty acids are found in oil-rich seeds and the oils extracted from them, such as corn, safflower, and soybean oils that are used in almost all snack foods and fast foods. Vegetable shortening, margarine, and partially hydrogenated oils also contribute to inflammatory pathways. Omega-3 fatty acids have an anti-inflammatory effect and are found in oily fish, walnuts, flaxseeds, hemp, and to a smaller degree in canola oils. The fats we get from our protein sources are also important; vegetable proteins (whole soy foods, beans, lentils, and other legumes) and fish and seafood are good substitutes for red meat in an "anti-inflammatory" diet.

How Stress Can Contribute to Inflammation and Cancer

Laboratory animal and human studies all suggest that key psychological factors, or stressors, can contribute to the development of cancer and influence the behavior of cancer once it occurs. Scientists believe that this is biologically related to an overstimulation of our *sympathetic* (fight or flight) nervous system, putting it out of balance with the *parasympathetic* (rest and digest) nervous system. Stressors disrupt the normal balance of hormones (including cortisol), triggering a stress response that turns on the "flight or fight" system. This triggers a chain of events that includes increases in our heart rate and blood pressure as well as biochemical changes, such as the formation of pro-inflammatory mediators that would be needed for injury or infection. Ideally, we would spend minimal time with our sympathetic nervous system on and the majority of time with the balancing force of the parasympathetic nervous system on, to help turn on the anti-inflammatory pathways that allow for healing, absorption of nutrients, and cell repair.

For most of us "feeling stressed" refers to an emotional feeling that is sometimes accompanied by the *physiological stress* response described above. In modern life, many ordinary daily activities, such as driving, trigger the "fight or flight" chain of events of physiological stress when no injury or infection needs to be dealt with. We often do not even feel stressed in these daily situations that require the quicker reflexes and multitasking ability that our sympathetic nervous system gives us, so we do not realize we need to "de-stress," or turn on the parasympathetic nervous system.

In women with ovarian cancer, depressed and anxious moods are associated with impairment of the normal immune response and an increase in tumor growth and cancer progression. In a study of mice with ovarian cancer, researchers found that chronic stress activated the "fight or flight" system and increased stress hormones, including cortisol and epinephrine (adrenaline). These hormones led to increased tumor growth and the development of new blood vessels around the cancer, improving its blood supply. In line with these findings, clinical studies have shown that the more social support someone has, the lower their blood concentration of growth factors (such as VEG-F, *vascular endothelial growth factor*), which stimulate vessel growth (known as *angiogenesis*), and inflammatory factors (such as IL-6, *interleukin-6*), which have been linked to worse ovarian cancer outcomes. Other studies have shown that the stress hormone norepinephrine influences tumor progression by modulating the factors implicated in angiogenesis and metastasis. In studies of people with a variety of cancers, this chain reaction of physiological stress has also been shown to decrease remission time and to allow the cancer to spread more quickly and aggressively compared with cancers in people who do not have chronic stressors.

Mind-Body Interventions for Stress

Several studies have shown that mind-body interventions can reverse some of the effects of ongoing stress on cancer. Mind-body interventions are thought to influence health by turning down our sympathetic nervous system and turning on our parasympathetic nervous system, thus turning down inflammation and the mediators of stress and inflammation. A mindfulness-based stress reduction (MBSR) program used a combination of yoga, guided imagery, home practice, group education, and skill building in a study of 90 people with a variety of cancers; they were either enrolled in an eight-week program (the study group) or placed on a wait list (the control group). For up to six months after the program, the participants in the program had improvements in mood and decreased stress compared with the wait-list group. Since this initial study, five additional trials with more than 400 participants demonstrated improvement in both mood and stress level using MBSR techniques. In a multicenter study of 410 mostly breast cancer patients using a program of breathing exercises, eighteen gentle yoga postures, and meditation, significant improvements were seen in sleep quality, fatigue, and overall quality of life.

Expressive techniques such as journaling and support groups have also shown benefits that are likely mediated by the mind-body connection. Sixty women with breast cancer participated in a trial exploring the benefit of journaling on cancer-related side effects; the women who kept a journal about traumatic events for 15 to 30 minutes a day for four days had decreased symptoms, fewer cancer-related medical visits, lower blood values of inflammatory markers, and immunological benefits that lasted for 4 to 8 months even with no further journaling. Hypnotherapy studies have shown decreases in anxiety and improvement in quality of life and general health measures. Spiritual well-being has been associated with decreases in anxiety, depression, discomfort, and isolation; better adjustment to the effects of cancer and cancer treatment; quicker recovery from treatment; and better health outcomes.

Although the research is limited for ovarian cancer survivors, given the significant potential for benefit and the low risk of harm, we recommend that you explore various mind-body interventions and find tools that work for you. A wide range of techniques have the potential to turn on our parasympathetic nervous system and turn down our stress response. All of the following are options to consider: laughter; prayer and other spiritual activities; creative outlets such as art, music, and dance; meditation; hypnosis and guided imagery (a state of relaxed and focused attention in which you concentrate on a feeling, idea, or suggestion to aid in healing); and biofeedback (using simple machines, people learn how to affect certain body functions that are generally beyond human awareness).

Using Integrative Approaches for Cancer-Related Symptoms

Numerous cancers and cancer-related symptoms are responsive to integrative approaches. In the largest study of massage therapy, researchers treated 1,290 cancer patients with Swedish massage, reflexology foot massage, or light touch massage and found significant improvements in multiple areas, including pain (improved by 48 percent), fatigue (43 percent), stress and anxiety (60 percent), nausea (51 percent), and depression (36 percent). In another trial that took place at multiple clinical sites, massage therapy was compared to simple touch in 380 adults with advanced cancer experiencing moderate to severe pain; results showed that just six 30-minute massage therapy sessions led to significant improvement in pain and mood. In a small study examining the effect of acupuncture on quality of life in women with advanced breast and ovarian cancer, researchers found significant benefits for pain, mood disturbances, and fatigue.

Sleep Disruption

A survey of women with ovarian cancer showed that the majority reported poor sleep quality, and almost half had used a sleep aid at least once in the prior month. Furthermore, disrupted sleep-wake cycles (circadian rhythms), night shift work, and exposure to light at night have all been shown to increase the risk of breast and perhaps other cancers. Sleep deprivation may directly contribute to cancer by stimulating inflammation, hindering damaged cells' ability to turn themselves off (apoptosis) and impairing cells' ability to repair DNA. The first approach we recommend to improve sleep quality and quantity is to focus on your *sleep hygiene*. Specific techniques include going to bed and getting up at the same time daily; establishing a consistent, relaxing bedtime routine; avoiding television and computer screens before bed; keeping your bedroom cool and dark; avoiding both caffeine after noon and alcohol before bed; and trying to dim your lights as the sun goes down. Integrative approaches such as guided imagery, deep breathing techniques, yoga, aromatherapy, and acupuncture may also be helpful. Herbs and supplements may be helpful: consider valerian, lemon balm, ashwagandha, and passion flower combinations; chamomile; or a sustained-release formulation of melatonin.

Insufficient melatonin, a hormone whose production is naturally stimulated by darkness and that regulates the sleep-wake cycle, is thought to be one of the links between lack of sleep and an increase in cancer risk, especially in hormone-related cancers such as breast and ovarian cancers. Melatonin has shown anti-estrogenic and anti-cancer properties. Multiple studies in different cancer types using relatively high doses of melatonin have shown some improvement in cancer outcomes and treatment-related side effects, but most of the studies have been small. One thing the studies clearly showed is that melatonin has relatively few side effects and is safe at high doses. Melatonin can be beneficial for sleep disruptions and has been shown to improve sleep quality and to decrease daytime sleepiness with fewer side effects than prescription medications. Currently, there is not enough evidence to recommend melatonin for ovarian cancer treatment, but in consultation with your physician, it should be considered if you are having trouble with sleep or have a history of disturbed circadian rhythms or night shift work.

Vasomotor Symptoms (Hot Flashes)

The cause of menopausal vasomotor symptoms (hot flashes) is unclear; disruption of the central thermoregulatory system in response to estrogen withdrawal is thought to play a part. For many ovarian cancer survivors, estrogen replacement may not be an option. There are, however, effective standard pharmacological approaches that your physician may suggest, including venlafaxine (a serotonin-norepinephrine reuptake inhibitor) and fluoxetine or citalopram (selective serotonin reuptake inhibitors). Successful integrative approaches to the symptoms of hot flashes include herbal supplements, dietary changes, acupuncture, mind-body techniques (guided imagery, hypnosis), aromatherapy, and exercise. The effectiveness of soy for hot flashes has not been proved, though there are studies showing improved blood cholesterol markers and support of good bone health. Flaxseeds are a good dietary source of lignans (phytoestrogens) and a rich plant source of omega-3 fatty acids. One small study showed that 2 tablespoons of ground flaxseed twice a day decreased the number of hot flashes by half and the intensity of hot flashes by 57 percent in the participants.

Several herbs have been studied and found to be safe for treating hot flashes. Black cohosh is not estrogenic; has no effects on serum sex hormone levels, vaginal epithelium, or endometrium; and is approved in Europe for the treatment of hot flashes. St. John's wort is widely used, either alone or with black cohosh, for hot flashes. St. John's wort is similar in action to the fluoxetine family and so has the same effect on speeding up the breakdown of other medications. A twelve-week study in women with menopausal symptoms found that 900mg of St. John's wort extract significantly improved psychological and physical symptoms and enhanced sexual well-being. Finally, there is a growing body of evidence for the effectiveness of acupuncture for the relief of hot flashes. In studies of acupuncture, the number and severity of hot flashes decreased, and participants had improvements in quality of life and overall sense of well-being.

Cancer-Related Fatigue and Chemo-Brain

Cancer-related fatigue (CRF) has been defined by the National Comprehensive Cancer Network (NCCN) as "a distressing, persistent, subjective sense of physical, emotional and/or cognitive tiredness or exhaustion related to cancer or cancer treatment that is not proportional to recent activity and interferes with usual functioning." CRF is more severe than the fatigue experienced by people who have not had cancer and does not get better with rest. Chemo-brain describes the cognitive changes associated with cancer and cancer treatment, most often experienced as difficulties with concentration, memory, multitasking, and planning ability. There seems to be an interrelationship between CRF and chemo-brain; similar interventions can help both conditions.

The etiologies of both CRF and chemo-brain are unclear; the effects of the cancer itself, inflammation, cancer treatments (chemotherapy, surgery, and radiation) are all possible contributors. Treatment of contributing factors such as dehydration, anemia, depression, anxiety, poor quality sleep, and pain can help both CRF and chemo-brain. Physical activity is the single most effective tool for both CRF and chemo-brain, providing significant benefits with as little as 30 minutes of activity five times a week. Integrative approaches that can help include massage, guided imagery, yoga, meditation, acupuncture, and herbal treatments. Supplements that can be considered after consultation with your physician include ashwagandha, astragalus, American ginseng, Asian ginseng, *Rhodiola rosea*, and *Bacopa*.

Nausea and Vomiting

Integrative modalities can be used for cancer-related and chemotherapy-related nausea and vomiting. Several large reviews of multiple studies have confirmed the benefit of acupuncture to treat postoperative nausea and vomiting and chemotherapy-induced nausea and vomiting. In the only trial examining women with ovarian cancer, 142 women receiving platinum-based chemotherapy got acupuncture, vitamin B_6, or both. The combination arm had the least nausea and vomiting. Although most studies do not show benefits of ginger tea, ginger capsules have been shown to be as good as the prescription drug metoclopramide for chemotherapy-related nausea and vomiting.

Conclusion

Integrative medicine encompasses the combination of conventional medicine with complementary medical practices for which there is evidence of safety and effectiveness. Trials that examine these practices specifically in ovarian cancer survivors are limited. Until more research can be performed, it is reasonable to extrapolate the results from some other studies to ovarian cancer survivors. A healthy and balanced diet, regular exercise, stress management, social support, regular sleep, and avoidance of tobacco have all shown benefits, with better cancer-related outcomes and enhanced quality of life. Numerous cancer and cancer-related symptoms are responsive to integrative approaches. For many areas, emerging data suggest that integrative interventions have positive effects:

- There is significant potential for benefit and low risk of harm for various mind-body interventions. We recommend that you explore and find tools that work for you to reduce stress, improve sleep, and address fatigue and vasomotor symptoms.
- Physical activity is the single most effective tool for both cancer-related fatigue and chemo-brain.
- An increasing number of trials suggest benefit to certain herbs and supplements, when used in the appropriate context. But remember, herbs and supplements have the potential for allergic reactions and can interact with over-the-counter and prescription medications. Talk with your oncologist or pharmacist before trying them.
- Whole foods remain the best way to get your nutrients and can provide safe, healthy, and delicious sources of nutrients that can support your well-being and improve your cancer outcomes.
- Just as it is important for you to discuss with your oncologist the risks and benefits of chemotherapy or surgery, you should examine the different aspects of complementary, alternative, and integrative medical treatments, and consider these treatments in the context of your current health and goals.

How we live matters.

A Personal Perspective on Image Recovery
Regina

I now have what ovarian cancer patients call a "front butt." These are created when you have open-abdominal surgery resulting in a fierce scar that runs from about mid-abdomen to the belly button, sometimes all the way to the pubic area. Then on either side of this scar are two new pouches of fat that hang like butt cheeks.

To go with this new butt, I have two new breasts created by implant reconstruction after a bilateral mastectomy. The new breasts also have scars. The one on the left is longer, as it leads to a pit in my excavated underarm. There are lines up the middle on both breasts to my new nipple tattoos, which are already fading after just two years. Heap on about 60 pounds, unruly hair, sparse eyebrows and eyelashes, and voila! You have an alien woman staring back at you from the mirror.

I am a four-year breast cancer and a three-year ovarian cancer survivor who has had ten surgeries and twelve rounds of chemotherapy. I am grateful to be alive, and to be NED [no evidence of disease]. I am not grateful for cancer's collateral damage.

When I was diagnosed with cancer, my main concern was getting the cancer out of my body as quickly as possible by any means possible. I had no idea the high price I'd pay for this. I am no longer the vibrant newlywed 52-year-old woman I was when I was diagnosed. My physical body and self-image are radically different. My sexual desire and capacity dried up (literally) after being put into surgical menopause. Then to seal the deal, I was put on an aromatase inhibitor, which causes hot flashes from hell and weight gain. My husband left me and took his health insurance with him. I haven't been able to work, and my financial status has gone from reasonably secure to precarious.

Now I am on an intense journey to create who I am as a woman, as a valuable member of society, and as something I never wanted to be: a cancer survivor. It has taken a lot of praying, reading, talking, and effort to get to where I am. Today, I stay mostly in a good place. I still have my sense of humor and my true friends. I still have my faith that there is something here for me to do.

I've been asked if I was glad I'd had cancer "because you learn what is really important." Ummm, no! I've always known what is important. I think what I've learned is what is important to *other* people, and I am grateful to be free from meaningless standards and expectations. I am more careful today about who I let occupy my time and space. Cancer took away two years of my life. I am determined not to give it more.

CHAPTER 10

Image Recovery

Paula J. Anastasia, RN, MN, AOCN

A fter a diagnosis of ovarian cancer or recurrent disease, most women will complete surgery and chemotherapy treatments and then be informed that there is no evidence of disease, or perhaps that the disease is stable or controlled. As described in chapter 13, a woman's disease "status" may be determined by physical exam, blood tests, imaging scans, or any combination of the three.

Although the news is good—you are told that you may resume your previous life, the life before it was interrupted by cancer—many women find a status of "no evidence of disease" or "stable or controlled disease" to be complicated and at times challenging. After all, they are not the same person they were, now having gone through the cancer journey. They certainly do not believe they look the same. A woman may find it hard to look in the mirror and see someone looking back at her whom she doesn't recognize. You, too, may not look like your familiar self, the one before cancer treatment. You possibly have little or no hair, your weight may have changed, you likely still feel tired, and now you are told to return to "normal." If you are returning to a workplace outside of the home, some of your colleagues assume that you will look the same, and they will expect your stamina to be similar to what it was before you took a work disability "vacation."

Yet ovarian cancer and its treatment affect more than a patient's physical self-image: they also insult her image of health, well-being, and mortality. They are an affront to the Whole Image, not simply the Visual Image. In this chapter we want to focus on image recovery in a global sense—the image recovery that occurs once the treatments are done and the disease is considered to be controlled or absent.

Recovery of the Visual Image

On a fairly predictable time line and in a fairly predictable way, most women who have had surgery and chemotherapy will eventually regain the physical appearance they had before treatment.

Hair, Nails, and Skin

Of the various aspects of recovery of the visual self, hair is the one you have the least control over. Your hair, fingernails, and skin will grow back on their own, and there isn't much you need to do to make sure this happens—although there are some things you can do to help your hair, fingernails, and skin recover from the trauma of treatment. Studies have shown that a fair amount can be done from a nutritional perspective to strengthen hair and keep it strong. Adequate nutrition, from vitamin supplements and food sources of protein, will help your hair and skin recover and make them stronger.

Every woman receiving a taxane chemotherapy, such as paclitaxel, will have hair loss from the head, in addition to possible loss of eyelashes, eyebrows, and body hair. Hair generally begins to regrow two months after the last chemotherapy infusion; it may take approximately six months for the hair to cover the head for a short chic hairdo. The texture of the new hair is usually different, perhaps gray and curly. Hair can be colored after chemotherapy, although the new hair may initially be more sensitive to hair dye. Tell your hairdresser about your treatment, in case there are more gentle products she or he recommends while the new hair is sprouting.

Studies support the use of hair rejuvenation agents such as Latisse and minoxidil. Minoxidil topical foam is approved for male pattern baldness but has shown some success in both genders after chemotherapy-related hair loss. Biosil is a brand name of orthosilicic acid, which as a supplement has shown to strengthen fine hair. Latisse is a prescription drug, approved to stimulate eyelash growth, and can be used after chemotherapy if the eyelashes appear to be sluggish in their regrowth. The medication is applied daily to the upper eyelids. The American Cancer Society offers support programs for appearance-related side effects.

Nail changes may occur as a result of various chemotherapy regimes. The nails may change color, become thin, peel, or break. If nails separate from the base or if fluid develops under the nails, it's essential to keep nails free of secondary infection. Local antibiotic ointments are helpful, as is soaking fingernails or toenails in a homemade solution consisting of equal parts white vinegar and tap water. If you think you might have an infection, consult your health care team or a dermatologist. The rate of nail growth is individualized. Vitamins such as biotin and Biosil have been documented to be helpful with nail growth. Of course, before taking any medications, even supplements, please talk with your health care team. Manicures, pedicures, and salon nail care are also permissible after chemotherapy, though you'll need to make sure that only clean, sterilized instruments are used on your nails. For thin nails, gel type manicures may keep nails protected longer than weekly manicures, although the gel removal process may be especially drying.

Many factors affect the condition of our skin: genetics, the environment, diet, medications, and cancer interventions such as surgery, chemotherapy, and radiation. Keeping skin free from infection is most important, especially if there are any open wounds, lesions, or sores on the body. Skin rashes may occur from specific chemotherapy, particularly liposomal doxorubicin. Skin changes and rashes may remain for several months, even when the chemotherapy treatments have been completed. Maintaining skin integrity with fragrance-free creams will retain moisture in the skin. When skin is too dry, it becomes itchy, which leads to scratching and possible infection. If skin is very flaky, an exfoliant cream can remove the dead skin. For cracks in skin, petroleum jelly, A&D ointment, or Desitin can serve as an effective barrier. Sunscreen and sun-protective clothing should be worn daily, especially when going outdoors.

Weight

Through a combination of being inactive and not taking in enough calories, people unfortunately lose weight in a manner that leads to loss of lean body mass (muscle) before loss of fat. What this means is that a patient who has been both inactive and nutritionally depressed will have lost a disproportionate amount of muscle mass. By contrast, some women will have no change in their ability to ingest calories and may even gain weight during their chemotherapy. Some women use food as a comfort but do not balance it with activity or exercise and therefore gain unwanted weight. A woman recovering from her ovarian cancer treatment needs more than just calories. Appropriate and aggressive nutritional support, which we talked about in chapter 6, is critical to maintaining a healthy weight and body mass index. Incorporating movement and exercise into your daily schedule is equally important.

Body Strength and Stamina

It is well known in the cancer community that diet and exercise may increase survival. Adding exercise as a goal to your daily routine may be very beneficial. If you were someone who exercised prior to your cancer diagnosis, this may not be a challenge for you. You may notice your stamina has decreased from before diagnosis, but resuming baseline goals is achievable. If you are not used to exercising daily, try adding some form of daily activity, whether you are walking in front of the house for 5 minutes or lifting soup cans as arm weights while watching television. Small segments of exercise are an improvement from no exercise at all. As you become comfortable with 5 to 10 minutes of exercise daily, you will notice an ability to increase to 15 to 30 minutes a day. Ideally, 60 minutes of activity is recommended; this can be divided into short segments throughout the day.

If you exercise too much or too fast or even too frequently, all you do is become sore and tired, and you lose the motivation to get out and exercise again. Remember two cardinal rules of exercise: first, be reasonable; and second, any exercise, as long as it causes no harm, is better than none.

There is another well-documented advantage of exercising: it makes you feel better. The endorphin release that comes from exercising is a good thing in many ways—ways that transcend the "feel good" effects. There are positive effects on blood flow to the essential body structures, as well as improved liver and kidney function. Exercise can also decrease fatigue and give you energy. That sounds like a contradiction, especially if you are too tired to exercise. Lack of exercise will cause muscle atrophy, or weakness, adding to the feeling of fatigue. Increasing activity will improve muscle strength and increase energy in the long term. Weight-bearing exercises will promote bone health and help to decrease the risk of osteoporosis. Weight-bearing exercises include standing, walking, bicycling, and running. Swimming is an excellent form of exercise but it is not considered weight bearing. Discuss with your practitioner the types of exercise best suited for your wellness, and ask whether a referral to a physical therapist or trainer would have benefit. Medications to supplement bone health, such as calcium, vitamin D_3, and a bisphosphonate, may also be recommended by your practitioner.

Recovery of Function

It is sometimes difficult to assess the functional state of an individual because there are two parts. The first is the percentage you think you are functioning at, compared to before your cancer diagnosis, and the second is how you would score your energy level. For instance, you can be going through the motions of all your day-to-day activities, household management, and working a job—thus, functioning at 80 to 90 percent—but your energy level may be only 60 percent because you have persistent fatigue.

It might be helpful to make lists of things that you need to do daily and determine which are important and which can be postponed or canceled. Many women have reported a new confidence in saying "no" once they have gone through the cancer journey. They have developed a healthier sense of self by doing only the things that matter, and saying "no," or "not at this time," to the other things. Recovery means physical and emotional wellness. Now is the time to make room for positive influences and energy, and to remove and disconnect from the negative and unpleasant acquaintances in your life. Stamina and energy may be improved and even restored by focusing on the positive events in your day. Maintaining adequate sleep is essential. If you are not able to fall asleep or stay asleep, or you are still tired in the morning, talk with your health care team to identify the cause of the sleep disturbance and how to get better sleep.

Fatigue may be due to many factors, including low blood counts from surgery or chemotherapy, lack of exercise, or depression. At the completion of chemotherapy, your blood counts, specifically your red count and white count, may return to "normal" within a couple of months, or in as long as a year. That does not mean that you won't be able to resume your baseline activities, but if you experience periods of fatigue, or less productive days, this is appropriate and expected. Patients and their family and friends need to keep in mind the long-term effects of chemotherapy treatments. Many patients want to return to "normalcy" and a productive life. This includes resuming family and role identities, whether as a daughter or a wife, a friend or an aunt, a mother or a grandmother. Those titles and roles are meaningful for many, many people.

In addition, many women have careers outside the home and are expected to return to that role, without any limitations. This is all achievable, but there will be times of doubt, when you feel overwhelming fatigue, and you will question whether you can maintain the same workload you had prior to your cancer treatment. Yes, you can. However, do allow yourself permission to need more time, and discuss with significant others if you want to reevaluate your choices. Many patients are more motivated than ever to resume their careers, while others want to re-examine what they want to do with the "rest of their life," knowing they have already survived a cancer diagnosis. There is no right or wrong in this scenario. There is only self-reflection.

A Personal Perspective on Taking Care of Social Needs

Marcie Paul

My only child was 12 years old when I was diagnosed with late-stage ovarian cancer, and she immediately became the focal point of my terror. Over time, however, she also fueled my strength, motivation, and salvation.

While terrified that she might grow up without a mother, I was nevertheless determined she'd somehow gain something positive from the horrific experience—how best to face adversity. It led me to a helpful revelation: I could not control *if* I had cancer, but I could control *how* I had cancer. This realization affected nearly everything going forward, from my ability to manage side effects and fear, to ultimately learning some inadvertent life lessons for us both.

I discovered it was important to find a balance between marching ahead without letting cancer define me or stop me from living fully, while still remaining open to those life-altering lessons. Primarily among them, I felt compelled to spend my time more purposefully. To take the cancer fight beyond my personal battle, I became a presenter in the Ovarian Cancer National Alliance's Survivors Teaching Students program, an advocacy leader and a grant reviewer for the U.S. Department of Defense's Ovarian Cancer Research Program. Because there wasn't an OCNA Partner Member in my state when I was diagnosed, I also became instrumental in developing one in Michigan. My daughter participated throughout, starting with a national fundraising walk in New York while I was still in treatment.

Today, she heads off to college with a level of maturity and social conscience she might not otherwise possess. And I not only continue to advocate on the state and federal levels for greater awareness, better access to care, and more research funding, but also volunteer as a patient mentor for MD Anderson Network and Jewish Family Service as well as Michigan Ovarian Cancer Alliance's Survivor-to-Survivor Support Network. I often share my view with them that advocacy is an extension of being a proactive, knowledgeable patient. Sometimes I also offer the tongue-in-cheek opinion that it's clearly self-serving because my life depends on it. But beyond truly believing that I am responsible for fighting this disease on the larger scale, it is also empowering, fulfilling, and healing. Additionally, it is profoundly gratifying to be able to give another teal sister some encouragement and hope. For me, helping others, whether through personal contact, organizational programs, or public policy, really seems to take some of the curse off the horror of living with cancer. I suspect my desire to be a role model for my daughter is one reason this is a significant part of my experience as a survivor.

CHAPTER 11

Taking Care of Social Needs

Paula J. Anastasia, RN, MN, AOCN

A cancer journey brings changes beyond the physical changes. Cancer can change a woman's relationships and roles with her spouse or significant other, and with her children and other family members. Some women find a new meaning to their life after going through cancer treatments. They are not happy that the cancer happened, but they find new purpose in their life and new value in the people they choose to share their time with. Trying to figure out why you got cancer may always remain elusive, but having had cancer may be the reason you renew your love for your family or your faith.

It can be liberating to say, "Life is short, and therefore I want to spend time only with people who are significant to me and who share my positive attitude." Life may look pristine because you are able to enjoy the present and appreciate the little things that in the past you may have overlooked or taken for granted. Knowing that you got through the surgery and chemotherapy may give you permission to slow down and think about yourself, perhaps for the first time in your life. For others, cancer does not bring a silver lining. Instead, cancer brings unpaid medical bills, isolation, fear, and more stressors. How each woman responds will be different and personal.

The reality of high health care costs, inadequate health care coverage, and daily bills can be overwhelming for many people. If you are employed outside the home and are provided health insurance through your employer, talk with your human resources department about insurance counseling, financial planning, and disability benefits. Find out about the Family and Medical Leave Act, a federal law that secures a job (sometimes without pay) when a person, including a family caregiver, needs to be away for medical reasons.

Many women who work outside the home find they want to return to their workplace setting because they appreciate the daily structure it offers—a distraction from their day-to-day cancer worries—and they value their colleagues as a social outlet. Disclosing your cancer diagnosis to your employer and coworkers can lead to self-doubt, especially if your job is physically demanding and you are not functioning at full capacity because of your chemotherapy side effects. Talk with your health care team about any acute or delayed limitations, during or after your treatment, that would interfere with working full or part time.

Your health care team can also provide referrals to people and organizations that can help with financial assistance and family assistance. There are advocacy groups in most cities, sometimes associated with a hospital, that provide excellent resources to patients who have a cancer diagnosis. In addition, you can contact any of the numerous online advocacy groups, such as the National Ovarian Cancer Coalition (NOCC), the Ovarian Cancer National Alliance (OCNA), Cancer Hope Network, and Cancer Care. If you live in a small town or rural area where there are no ovarian cancer–specific support groups, there may be a breast cancer or general women's cancer support group, which can provide friendship, networking, and suggestions for treatment-related assistance with transportation, childcare services, and financial resources.

Some women feel vulnerable when their physician tells them they are in remission and they can now extend their follow-up exam to every three months instead of every month. They may be surprised to find that they feel insecure when they finish chemotherapy and have a new worry that the cancer will recur. Patients often describe the health care team as their safety net, and now being away from the cancer center may cause anxiety. When they finish treatment, many patients ask, "What do I do now?" and "How do I know if the cancer is coming back?" Initially, patients worry that every ache and discomfort in the body is new cancer. Trying to return to normal and find the new normal will take time. Making plans, celebrating today, and setting new goals for the future is how many women approach their tomorrow.

Adjusting to life after cancer and the uncertainty of a recurrence, or perhaps living with a chronic disease because the ovarian cancer has already recurred, can cause free-floating anxiety, which in turn can cause alienation and suffering. Alienation and suffering sometimes include depression and anxiety, which are medical conditions that can be treated. The patient, family, and caregivers must acknowledge the patient's feelings and work together to cope with her fear, which may feel paralyzing—so much so that she is not able to move forward with decision making. Although every person will respond and cope differently, there are healthy and unhealthy coping behaviors. The opportunity to talk to another cancer survivor within a support group, or to a "buddy patient" introduced to the patient by the health care team, can help validate your feelings. Hearing that someone else has gone through a similar treatment and has felt what you are feeling can be very reassuring, and talking with other patients about how they successfully overcame their fears can help you overcome yours. You might also ask for a referral to a social worker or therapist (a psychologist or psychiatrist), or your doctor may recommend one, to help your emotional wellness.

Many women with ovarian cancer have a close physician-nurse-patient relationship stemming from the chronic nature of the disease. If your health care team has not inquired about your emotional health and social needs, you can start the conversation. Psychological health is as much a part of your wellness as physical health.

Family and Friends

During times of real or even perceived crisis, family structures and interpersonal relationships are put to the test, and their strengths or weaknesses become evident. Relationships with friends, coworkers, and acquaintances will be re-evaluated at such times. When friends and family say, "Call me if you need anything," it does add another responsibility for you to own. But most people who say that really do want to be of service. Most often, they feel helpless or don't know what to do. So, *give* them tasks, whether picking up groceries, driving you to a doctor's appointment, or doing a load of laundry. It will make both of you feel better, to be able to give and receive kindness.

Some women who have been diagnosed with ovarian cancer may try to maintain their independence and use control as a coping mechanism. They may say that they don't want to be perceived as a burden to their spouse, or to see their children's school or daily schedule interrupted. Even though the focus is on the woman who has the diagnosis of ovarian cancer, other parts of her life will also be affected. The cancer journey can affect the entire family unit. Spouses often are supportive and compassionate, but they may also be overly protective. If they feel they have no control over a situation, they may focus more on their work or career. School-age kids may display behavioral changes such as regression to a younger age or clingy behavior. Older children may exhibit changes in schoolwork. Talking together as a family, discussing what will change and what will stay the same, can help the family adapt and provide some reassurance that the unit will remain intact. Family support groups or individual counseling have benefited many families and individuals, and they provide a safe venue for sharing feelings.

Some women fear they won't be desirable to their partner as a result of surgical and chemotherapy side effects. For single women, the fear of disclosure in a potential new relationship, and a concern about who would want them now that they have had ovarian cancer, may prevent a woman from moving forward with social relationships. These are very common and normal feelings that women with ovarian cancer may experience at various times during their cancer journey. Do remember that relationships begin with friendship and trust. It is not necessary to reveal all your health information on a first date. Most people have some private or family issues that they would rather not divulge to a first-time acquaintance. For example, what about a sexually transmitted disease? Unless you are having sexual relations that day, it is reasonable to wait until there is trust and the need to share this information. What if you have had financial trouble, bankruptcy, or a family member who has broken the law? You may meet a potential partner who has similar hesitation about when to overshare. Friendship, trust, and companionship begin a relationship. Not surprisingly, there will be people who care about you as a whole person, and their character is what will define them to you.

The interpersonal relationship between you and your significant other may be challenged if there was tension prior to your cancer diagnosis. Not everyone has healthy or appropriate coping skills. Unfortunately, the additional dynamic of a cancer diagnosis added to a fragile relationship may be enough to break the formerly supportive temperament of the partner. On the other hand, relationships that are secure and strong prior to a cancer diagnosis often become stronger through the cancer journey. Of course, not every day will be pleasant or easy, but fully appreciating the most important person in your life and not taking that person for granted occupies a place high up on the importance list. Life after cancer may not be the same; it may be different, it may be uncertain, it may be better. For some women and their families, meeting with a relationship or family therapist may be helpful in talking about the new normal after ovarian cancer treatment.

Self-advocacy is a term for empowering a person to define her priorities and take the initiative with her health care team to manage and improve her individual needs. Self-advocacy can include managing side effects, finding and using help to support emotional and psychological adjustment, and striving for social well-being. In self-advocacy, patients seek knowledge, improve decision-making skills, and practice self-reflection. The patient's journey through a cancer diagnosis and treatment can cause an evolution of strength in becoming an advocate for herself.

Sexuality

Sexual health is often overlooked as a factor in the quality of life of someone who is dealing with a life-threatening illness such as ovarian cancer. Not everyone is interested in maintaining a sexual relationship, but when asked, most people are still interested in intimacy. Sexuality is a physical, mental, and social connection to another human being. Intimacy can include the feeling of being in a close personal relationship that includes the physical, emotional, mental, and spiritual connection. It does not require the act of sex. It can just include touching, hugging, or cuddling.

Ovarian cancer surgery can affect self-esteem and can change a woman's image of her body because of scars, weight loss or gain, and other changes. Women are often concerned that sex will hurt, because of their recent surgery, a surgically induced menopause, or vaginal dryness, and they wonder if they will be able to have an orgasm. Finding a comfortable position, or using pillows for support, may alleviate pain. There may be some vaginal dryness postsurgery, requiring generous amounts of lubrication before vaginal intercourse. The loss of estrogen, caused by natural menopause or surgically induced menopause, will cause vaginal thinning and dryness. Lubricants and vaginal moisturizers, both available over the counter, will diminish the discomfort. If a woman was able to achieve an orgasm before the surgery, then orgasm is possible postsurgery.

Sexually speaking, the most common change is a decrease in libido. This change can be a result of estrogen deficiency from removal of ovaries, chemotherapy treatments, or side effects such as pain, fatigue, or nausea. Even after these side effects resolve, women may still report low libido. Medications such as antidepressants and narcotics can also decrease libido. In addition, vaginal dryness can cause discomfort with vaginal intercourse, and that physical discomfort contributes to the lack of arousal and decreased sexual satisfaction. Over-the-counter non-estrogen vaginal moisturizers can be applied into the vagina simply, using an applicator, weekly or several times a week. These moisturizers will decrease the vaginal irritation caused by vaginal thinning, although they will not reverse the effects. Vaginal lubricants, also sold over the counter, will still be needed before vaginal intercourse, even if using a vaginal moisturizer. In women for whom vaginal intercourse is not an option, other forms of sexual pleasure include oral or manual stimulation. In individual cases, vaginal estrogen may be indicated and prescribed by your health care practitioner; vaginal estrogen can reverse the vaginal thinning, or atrophy, that results from lack of estrogen.

The question remains of how to get in the mood. For couples who want to be sexually intimate, planning or scheduling a date is the most practical way to set the mood. Knowing ahead of time that you and your partner want to have sex on a specific date and time allows both partners to prepare emotionally and mentally and will help build excitement. You have time for getting ready, whether this involves wearing particular clothing to make you feel attractive, wearing a head covering or wig, setting the mood and location, or using candles or low lighting. Some couples enjoy adult toys or movies. Whatever is agreed on between two individuals determines what is appropriate. If you have any residual side effects such as pain or nausea, plan your medication an hour prior to your date. If you need to schedule a nap or rest period earlier in the day, plan that too.

There is no reason you can't make your sexual relationship satisfying and romantic, even if you plan it in advance. For some women or couples, a referral to a sexual health expert is beneficial. Techniques that have been suggested include touch therapy, in which the couple takes turns touching each other's body, such as neck, breasts, and inner thigh, and communicating which sensations feel better. As people age, sensory and touch receptors may change, so what used to feel pleasurable may no longer elicit the same response. Therefore, rediscovering what turns each other on begins with communicating with your partner. Talking with your health care team together with your partner is a valuable way to help reduce fears and misinformation, so that sexuality can be a part of your return to wellness.

A Personal Perspective on Genetic Testing

Carey Fitzmaurice

In January 2006 I found out that cousins of mine in the United Kingdom, sisters who had both had breast cancer in their thirties, had been part of a study that identified a new BRCA mutation. I had just started to look into getting tested myself when I was diagnosed with Stage IIIC ovarian cancer. We proceeded with my initial treatment with the assumption that I was BRCA+, which later testing proved.

At the time, there was less information about what a BRCA+ ovarian cancer survivor should do about breast cancer risk. I decided that I did not want to have cancer again, and I sought a prophylactic mastectomy. I was turned down by the first surgeon I saw. By the time I had things set with another surgeon, my ovarian cancer had recurred, so I put off surgery. Unfortunately, a few months later, I was diagnosed with Stage IIB breast cancer.

I've also been the beneficiary of treatments shown to be more effective in BRCA+ patients. I know that more of these targeted therapies are coming.

I am among the oldest of my generation of cousins from the branch of my family with the mutation, which comes from my father's father's father. Most of my female relatives who could be at risk have been tested, and most have been positive. I stay away from the younger women's decision making concerning what to do next, although I am a living example. We have been found by some long-lost cousins because they have been searching for more family to flesh out their family medical histories.

I do a lot of ovarian cancer advocacy work. My take on it always involves the genetic component. Doctors need education, not only that first surgeon I went to, but also those who still tell patients that you can't inherit the mutation from your father. Also, BRCA is known as the "breast cancer gene," and too many women who know, via family history, that they might be at risk for breast cancer have no idea that ovarian cancer needs to be considered as well.

Even those who have already been diagnosed should be tested. Not only can they prevent a second primary cancer, but their treatment could be different, with more and more new drugs that are most effective when the mutation is present.

A genetic counselor, especially one who has experience with BRCA, should be considered an important part of an oncology team.

CHAPTER 12

Genetic Testing

Elizabeth A. Wiley, MS, CGC, and Kala Visvanathan, MD

Diagnosis of ovarian cancer often elicits questions regarding cancer risk. A woman may wonder why she developed ovarian cancer, or she may wonder if she is at an increased risk for other cancers due to this diagnosis. There may be concerns about whether her children or siblings are at a higher risk for developing cancer as well. Genetic testing is a tool that can often provide information regarding cancer risks for a patient and her family members, which makes it possible for health care providers to recommend more personalized screening and preventive measures to manage these risks. In approximately 20 percent of women who have ovarian cancer, a genetic change can be identified that explains their diagnosis of ovarian cancer.

Genetics Introduction

A gene is a section of DNA (deoxyribonucleic acid) that provides instructions to build and maintain the cells of your body. Genes control how each cell in your body functions, including how often each cell divides and how long each cell lives. Genes are also responsible for the passing of traits from generation to generation. For example, genes determine your eye color, blood type, and susceptibility to disease. They do so by making substances called proteins that perform specialized actions in your body. Genes provide the instructions, and proteins carry out these instructions.

Every person has approximately twenty-five thousand different genes within each one of his or her cells. Most genes are present in pairs, and we all have two copies of almost every one of our genes. One set of this gene pair is inherited from our mother, and the other set of this gene pair is inherited from our father.

A *mutation* is a variation in the makeup of a gene that can cause it not to work properly. A mutation on a gene can lead to the production of an abnormal protein or no protein at all, which in turn stops the cell from functioning properly. Cancer comes about because of an accumulation of mutations in many genes within a cell over time. For example, if there is a mutation on a gene that causes the cell to divide more rapidly than it is supposed to, or to live longer than it should, the cells with that mutation can grow out of control, and cancer can develop.

Gene mutations can be classified as *somatic* or *germline*. Somatic means "of the body," and somatic mutations refer to changes that occur in the genes in a specific cell or group of cells; however, we are not born with these mutations, and they are not present in every cell in the body. It is not always clear exactly what causes somatic mutations to occur, though environmental exposures, such as tobacco use and ultraviolet (UV) radiation, as well as age play significant roles. Somatic mutations happen in our cells all the time, and the body is able to repair many somatic gene mutations before they are able to cause a problem. However, sometimes the damage is too great, and mutations accumulate, allowing the cell to grow and divide uncontrollably. Such uncontrolled growth and division can lead to cancer development.

By comparison, inherited mutations are in the germline, which means that they are present in the DNA of every cell of the body, including the eggs and sperm. Because germline mutations are present in these reproductive cells, this type of gene mutation can be passed from generation to generation. Hereditary ovarian cancer occurs when an individual is born with a mutation on a gene that controls cell growth and division (*tumor suppressor gene*) or on a gene that repairs DNA mistakes (mismatch repair gene). A person who has a germline mutation in a tumor suppressor gene has impaired control over these processes, and a person who has a germline mutation in a mismatch repair gene has a higher chance for developing somatic gene mutations that can lead to cancer.

The majority of ovarian cancer diagnoses are sporadic, which means they occur in the absence of a family history and are due to an accumulation of somatic mutations over time. Many people are surprised to hear that germline mutations that predispose a person to cancer development are uncommon, and only about 20 percent of all ovarian cancers are due to an inherited germline mutation.

Inheritance

An important concept to understand about hereditary ovarian cancer is its inheritance pattern. How are gene mutations passed through families? If someone has a gene mutation, what is the risk for family members to have that same mutation?

All currently known hereditary causes of ovarian cancer are inherited in an *autosomal dominant* manner. *Autosomal* means that these genetic mutations are not sex-specific; both women and men are equally likely to inherit and pass on mutations that are located on genes related to hereditary ovarian cancer. *Dominant* means that having a mutation on only one of the two gene copies is enough to cause a higher risk for cancer. Thus, if a parent has a gene mutation, each offspring will have a 50 percent chance of inheriting that gene mutation (and have the associated higher risk for cancer) and a 50 percent chance of not inheriting the gene mutation. Those who do not have a gene mutation that causes a higher risk for cancer cannot pass the mutation on to their children.

Inheriting a mutation on a gene associated with cancer does not mean that an individual will definitely develop cancer in his or her lifetime. Rather, these gene mutations place individuals at a higher risk for developing cancer. A person may have inherited a mutation that puts him or her at higher risk for developing cancer but may never go on to develop cancer. This concept is called *reduced penetrance*. Why some people with a gene mutation develop cancer while others do not is not well understood; it is likely due to some interaction of genes and environmental exposures, as well as lifestyle factors, many of which are unknown. What's important is that, regardless of whether someone with a gene mutation develops cancer, there is still a 50 percent chance for that person's offspring to inherit the mutation.

Genetic Counseling for Hereditary Ovarian Cancer

Genetic testing for hereditary cancer syndromes can be a difficult landscape to navigate. It is a constantly evolving field, and it can be difficult to process and understand all the information associated with inherited cancer risks. Should you have genetic testing, and if so, what testing is recommended? What types of test results can you get, and what would those results mean for the health of you and your family members? Because of the complexities of genetic testing, and because it is important for patients to understand the benefits and limitations of genetic testing, we recommend that patients interested in testing pursue a consultation with a multidisciplinary clinical cancer genetics service for genetic counseling and clinical management recommendations.

Genetic counseling is a process that includes a variety of elements. Your medical and family histories will be assessed to determine the chance of a hereditary cancer syndrome in your family, and you will receive education about genetic testing, inheritance, and management recommendations as well as counseling to help you make informed decisions regarding genetic testing and cancer risk management.

Protection against Genetic Discrimination

Many families are concerned about how genetic testing may affect their ability to obtain and maintain insurance policies. Genetic discrimination is the misuse of genetic information, either by insurance companies to increase premiums or discontinue coverage, or by employers to determine an individual's employability. To help allevi-ate concerns regarding discrimination related to genetic testing, the Genetic Information Nondiscrimination Act (GINA) was signed into law in May 2008.

GINA prohibits insurers in both the group and the individual health insurance markets from requiring genetic testing or using genetic information to determine eligibility or establish premiums. GINA does not apply to the Tricare Military Health System, the Vet-erans Administration, the Indian Health Service, or the Federal Em-ployees Health Benefits plans. However, these groups have their own internal policies in place to protect against insurance discrimination. GINA's protections do not apply to life insurance, disability insurance, or long-term care insurance. Although many states have laws that provide some level of protection for these types of coverage, there is no protection from discrimination on the federal level for these plans.

Regarding genetic discrimination in the workplace, GINA pro-hibits employers with more than fifteen employees from requiring genetic testing or using genetic information to make hiring or pro-motional decisions, or to determine eligibility for training programs. Similar to its insurance protections, GINA's employment safeguards do not extend to members of the U.S. military or employees of the federal government. A separate law, passed in 2000, offers protection to federal employees from discrimination in employment. The U.S. military has its own policies in place that may protect members of the military from genetic discrimination.

Gathering Family History Information

At this stage, your family history is one of the most important tools that can be used to assess cancer risk. Your family cancer his-tory provides information that is useful in determining whether there is a hereditary cancer syndrome in your family, and if so, what syn-drome might be present. This information can help guide your health care provider in ordering and interpreting genetic testing. Even when genetic testing is not indicated, or when genetic testing is performed but a mutation is not identified, your family medical history can pro-vide useful information regarding what other cancers you or your family members may be at risk for. Therefore, it is important to gather as much information about your family's health history as you can. Keep in mind that because you inherit 50 percent of your genes from your mother and 50 percent from your father, both your maternal and paternal family histories of cancer are important.

To start gathering your family's health history, it is often easiest to start with close family members (children, siblings, and parents), and then move on to more distant family members (aunts, uncles, and grandparents). Gather as much of the following information as possible when collecting your family's health history:

- Ethnicity, race, or your family's country of origin
- Approximate year of birth for each family member (for example: 1950s)
- For relatives who have passed away:
  - How old were they when they passed away?
  - What was the cause of death?
- For relatives who were diagnosed with cancer:
  - How old were they when they were first diagnosed?
  - From what organ did the cancer originate?
- For all relatives: history of surgeries, especially removal of the uterus (hysterectomy) or ovaries (oophorectomy)
- For all relatives: history of colon polyps
- For all relatives: lifestyle factors, such as exercise habits; hobbies; diet; and alcohol, tobacco, or other drug use

If possible, it is always helpful to have medical records or death certificates that can clarify, confirm, or provide details about a family member's medical history. Learn everything you are able to, with the understanding that you will not be able to collect complete information about all your relatives.

It may be difficult to know where to begin gathering this information. There are several online resources available that provide guidance on how to obtain and document family medical history. Frequently, the best way to start is by simply talking to your family members. Family history information is often shared at family get-togethers, such as reunions or holiday dinners, and the Surgeon General has even declared Thanksgiving to be National Family History

Day. It may also be helpful to pursue a one-on-one conversation with specific family members to obtain a more complete record of what they know. Often, older relatives such as parents or grandparents are a good source of information. Important: keep a written record of these conversations that you can refer back to.

You may feel hesitant to ask your family members about their personal medical histories. Certainly, some relatives may not wish to share their medical information, and their boundaries must be respected. You may be surprised, however, to find that most of your relatives are willing to share their health history, especially if they understand that this knowledge will be beneficial to their family's health. Figures 12.1 and 12.2 show examples of family trees, a structure you might find helpful in keeping track of your family medical history.

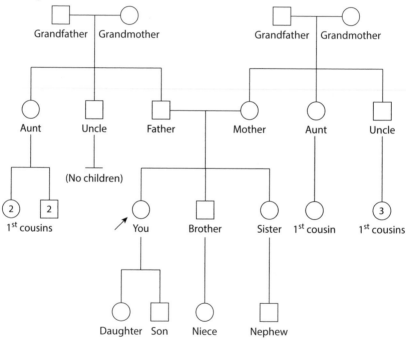

 = Male/boy

◯ = Female/girl

FIGURE 12.1   Example of a family tree.

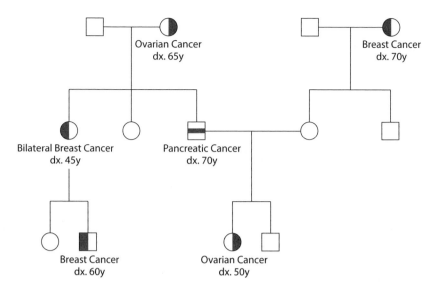

FIGURE 12.2   Example of a family tree showing hereditary breast and ovarian cancer due to a BRCA mutation. Circles = females, squares = males, right-sided shading = ovarian cancer, left-sided shading = breast cancer, middle shading = other type of cancer.

Syndromes Associated with Hereditary Ovarian Cancer

Once you have gathered your family history information, a specialist can review your personal and family history to assess what genetic testing, if any, would be helpful for you and your family. Researchers have identified the genes that are responsible for the majority (>90 percent) of hereditary ovarian cancer. However, some causes of inherited ovarian cancer remain unexplained.

BRCA1 and BRCA2 Hereditary Breast and Ovarian Cancer

BRCA1 and BRCA2 are tumor suppressor genes. As with all genes, every person has two copies of each. When functioning properly, BRCA1 and BRCA2 protect the body from tumor development. Individuals who are born with a mutation on one of these two genes, however, have a significantly higher lifetime risk for developing different types of cancer, including hereditary breast and ovarian cancer (HBOC).

The general risk for a woman in the United States to develop ovarian cancer in her lifetime is less than 1 in 71; factors affecting this risk were addressed earlier in this book (see chapter 1). In contrast, women who are born with a germline mutation on BRCA1 or BRCA2 have a 10 to 45 percent lifetime risk for developing epithelial ovarian cancer. Approximately 15 percent of women who are diagnosed with epithelial ovarian cancer have a germline BRCA1 or BRCA2 mutation. Women with a BRCA1 or BRCA2 mutation also have an elevated risk for developing breast cancer that is estimated to be between 40 and 87 percent over a lifetime. Mutations in BRCA1 and BRCA2 also confer an increased risk for prostate and breast cancer in men, as well as a modestly increased risk for other cancers, such as melanoma and pancreatic cancer, in both men and women.

Although only a small percentage of women with ovarian cancer carry a mutation on one of these genes, it is important to identify women who may be carriers of this mutation. Identification of a BRCA1 or BRCA2 mutation allows us to assess a patient's future cancer risks; if a woman has been diagnosed with ovarian cancer, is she at significantly increased risk for developing breast cancer? Importantly, it also allows us to offer predictive testing to a patient's at-risk family members, to assess their cancer risk. In many cases, family members who do not carry the identified mutation have a cancer risk that is closer to the risk in the general population and can therefore follow population guidelines for cancer surveillance. The family members who are found to carry the same mutation, however, are known to be at higher risk for cancer and can be offered preventive surgeries and increased surveillance to help mitigate the increased risks for breast and ovarian cancer.

Several characteristics about a patient's medical and family histories can help us to identify who is at a higher risk for carrying a mutation on BRCA1 or BRCA2—and who may therefore benefit from genetic testing.

- High-grade serous ovarian cancer. The majority of ovarian cancers diagnosed in women with a BRCA1 or BRCA2 mutation are of high-grade serous histology.

- Breast cancer and epithelial ovarian cancer in the same woman.
- Cancers diagnosed at younger ages. Generally, this means cancers diagnosed younger than the age of 50.
- Multiple family members spanning multiple generations who are affected with breast or ovarian cancer.
- A family history of male breast cancer or pancreatic cancer.
- Ashkenazi Jewish ethnicity. Although BRCA1 and BRCA2 mutations are found in all ethnic populations, these mutations are ten times more common in individuals of Ashkenazi Jewish descent.

Lynch Syndrome

Lynch syndrome is an inherited condition that causes a significantly increased lifetime risk for colorectal cancer. Thus, it is classified as a hereditary colon cancer syndrome, and it is also referred to as hereditary nonpolyposis colorectal cancer syndrome (HNPCC). However, Lynch syndrome also confers an increased risk for other cancers, including ovarian cancer, and the Lynch syndrome accounts for approximately 3 percent of all ovarian cancers. The syndrome is caused by germline mutations in mismatch repair genes, which are normally responsible for repairing somatic mutations in the DNA. We currently know of six mismatch repair genes that explain most cases of Lynch syndrome; these genes are called MLH1, MSH2, MSH6, PMS1, PMS2, and MLH3. However, mutations in MLH1 and MSH2 are responsible for 70 percent of the cases of Lynch syndrome.

When the data are combined, men and women with Lynch syndrome have up to an 80 percent lifetime risk for colorectal cancer. When the data are separated by sex, however, men have up to a 90 percent lifetime risk, while women have a 60 percent lifetime risk. The second most common cancer seen in Lynch syndrome is endometrial cancer. Women with Lynch syndrome have up to a 60 percent lifetime risk for this cancer, which means that these women have as high of a risk for endometrial cancer as they have for colorectal cancer.

Like testing for HBOC, testing for Lynch syndrome is not appropriate for all women. Features in the medical and family history allow us to identify patients for whom Lynch syndrome testing is appropriate:

- A family history of colorectal or endometrial cancer, especially cancers diagnosed younger than 50 years of age
- An individual who has been diagnosed with multiple primary Lynch-related cancers
- Multiple family members spanning multiple generations affected with Lynch-related cancers

As with mutations on BRCA1 and BRCA2, identifying a mutation on a Lynch syndrome–related gene can provide important information regarding cancer risks for a patient and her family members. Individuals with Lynch syndrome should undergo frequent colon cancer screening, and it is generally recommended that people who have Lynch syndrome undergo colonoscopy every year to screen for colon cancer. It might also be recommended that they undergo regular endoscopic surveillance of their upper gastrointestinal tract (the stomach and small intestine). Women with Lynch syndrome who have not had a hysterectomy or bilateral salpingo-oophorectomy should also be offered surveillance and preventive surgeries to manage endometrial cancer risk, and may be offered these for ovarian cancer risk. Finally, specific blood and urine tests should be performed annually to screen for the other cancers associated with Lynch syndrome.

Peutz-Jeghers Syndrome

Peutz-Jeghers syndrome (PJS) is a rare condition caused by mutations on the STK11 gene that confers an increased risk for benign and malignant tumors of the gastrointestinal tract, breast, ovary, cervix, and testes. People with PJS develop a unique type of polyp in their gastrointestinal tract, and they also develop distinct freckles on their face, hands, and feet. Unlike HBOC and Lynch syndrome, which are typically associated with epithelial ovarian cancers, women with PJS are at higher risk for a non-epithelial ovarian tumor called a *sex-cord tumor with annular tubules* (SCTAT). This type of tumor is usually benign, though it has the potential to become malignant.

Often, a diagnosis of PJS can be made by clinical assessment of an individual's health and family histories. If genetic testing is performed and a STK11 mutation is identified, predictive genetic testing would be available to family members, and increased cancer surveillance for the malignancies associated with PJS is available to those who are found to have this condition.

Recent Developments in Hereditary Ovarian Cancer

The three syndromes discussed in this chapter account for more than 90 percent of inherited causes of ovarian cancer. Yet some patients who have characteristics suggestive of hereditary ovarian cancer (for example, young-onset cancer or a strong family history of ovarian cancer) do not have an identifiable mutation on any of these genes. Therefore, some groups are focusing their research on finding new genes that may be related to ovarian cancer risk.

Thankfully, some progress has been made as a result of this research, and scientists have discovered other genes that appear to be associated with ovarian cancer risk. Germline mutations on genes, such as Rad51C, Rad51D, and BRIP1, appear to explain the cancer history in a small percentage of families that have many members with ovarian cancer but no HBOC- or Lynch-associated gene mutation. Germline mutations have been found in some women who have a personal history of ovarian cancer but no family history of cancer. It is believed that many of these genes also exhibit reduced penetrance, meaning that although they are passed on genetically from one generation to the next, they have a lower likelihood of resulting in cancer. Much work still needs to be done to understand the cancer risks that are associated with mutations on these genes so that appropriate screening recommendations can be established.

Sometimes, even after careful assessment, it is not clear which one syndrome may be responsible for a woman's personal and family histories of cancer. There is occasionally overlap in how these syndromes appear in families, or the pattern of cancer in a family may not look like any one known syndrome. Therefore, some women may receive a recommendation to undergo testing for a panel of many genes that are related to ovarian cancer risk. Performing testing using a gene panel can be beneficial under the correct circumstances; however, interpreting the results produced by this type of testing can be difficult. Because of this difficulty, testing for a panel of genes is not currently recommended for every woman with a diagnosis of ovarian cancer.

Genetic testing for hereditary ovarian cancer is a valuable tool that can be used to classify and manage cancer risk within families. There is still much left to learn, however. Because the field of cancer genetics is rapidly evolving, it's best to maintain contact with your health care providers, who can help you keep up to date with advances in this field.

A Personal Perspective on Therapy Completion and Surveillance

Susan Leighton

The airplane door opened, and the jumpmaster gave me a push as I stood trembling with fear when I realized I had no parachute. That is the exact feeling I had the day my gynecologic oncologist said, "Chemo is over; you are in remission. See you in three months." For the previous four months I had been in constant contact with the doctor, his nurse practitioner, or the nurses in the chemotherapy unit. Now I was supposed to walk among healthy people praying that the remission would last. How would I manage without a weekly call telling me my CA-125 was still down or without the frequent check-ins with the doctor? During those first three months, every twinge of pain was a sign to me that the cancer was back. I even took to measuring my abdominal girth when I felt a little bloated, forgetting that I had eaten way too much. My family and friends were constantly reminding me that it was gone and that I needed to live. They had a tough time understanding why I could not just let it go. My CA-125 was 17 at the end of chemo, and I obsessed when the number went to 24 only to have it return to 17 three months later. I begged my doctor for a scan many times during those first few months until one day I awoke and found the worry was loosening its grip.

Eighteen months into remission, my CA-125 started trending up: 29, 45, 120 . . . I heard the enemy approaching at an alarming rate. Scans did not show any disease. I took a leap of faith with my GYN/oncologist and decided to not treat the number and wait for symptoms to develop or imaging to show evidence of cancer. Maybe having learned to deal with the anxiety during the past eighteen months helped me navigate this "watch and wait approach." I went from knowing I was in remission to knowing it was growing and being monitored every three months. Was it easy? No, but it was the best option for me.

It was another seven and a half years before I started having symptoms. My CA-125 reached 950, and a PET scan showed a huge tumor in my chest. A cardiothoracic surgeon removed the tumor, and within six weeks my CA-125 was 7, where it has been for the last nine years. Once again I was shoved out the plane door and out into the world of infrequent blood tests and visits to my doctor. Anxiety never disappears, but it does lessen over time. One day I noticed that I had not thought about the cancer for several days. A window was opening, and life was spilling back in, replacing the anxiety. Sure, I still think about it when I lose a friend to the disease or for a few days before or after my annual visits to the GYN/oncologist, but there are far more days when I don't give it a minute of my time.

CHAPTER 13

Therapy Completion and Surveillance

Ritu Salani, MD, MBA

After therapy has been completed, one may expect things to go back to normal. The transition to life after treatment can be difficult, however. Many patients feel lost, partly because there are longer intervals between doctor visits. Patients may also experience an overwhelming feeling of "Now what?" The somewhat abrupt change from close and repeated contact with medical providers to the end of therapy and the beginning of surveillance can lead to anxiety. It may also lead to interruptions in follow-up care.

To make this transition seamless, the Institute of Medicine, which works to improve health and health policy, created a report entitled *From Cancer Patient to Cancer Survivor: Lost in Transition.* The report provides recommendations for this time frame and covers a wide range of issues, including follow-up care, prevention of new and recurrent cancer, and the management of cancer and therapy side effects. A patient who is able to anticipate the changes in her care after treatment is completed is less likely to be anxious. This chapter reviews recommendations for what to do and how to "be" after treatment is completed.

First, after completion of therapy, you should ask your provider to tell you the status of your cancer and what the status means in regard to the risk of the cancer coming back (recurrence). Your cancer team might use one of the following terms to describe a cancer that is not detectable, which is typically the case after primary therapy has been completed: no (clinical) evidence of disease, also referred to as NED; (clinical) remission; or complete (clinical) response. The term *clinical* implies that the status is based on your symptoms, examination, and tumor markers (if applicable). Though the term *cure* also fits in this category, it is not often used because it implies that the risk of the cancer coming back is low to none. Although cure is the goal and the hope of therapy, ovarian cancer, unfortunately, has a high risk of recurrence (which is discussed in more detail below).

Your cancer team may use one of the next set of terms if there is still disease present. These terms are often more appropriate when dealing with recurrent disease, but they may also be used to describe status during or after initial treatment. Partial response is when the disease has reduced by 30 percent in size and there are no new lesions. Progressive disease describes a 20 percent increase in size or the presence of new tumor lesions. Stable disease is used when the disease status does not meet criteria to be considered progressive or partial response. These terms indicate that cancer is still detectable and often imply that additional or different treatments might be required.

Surveillance

Though treatment is often the most talked about part of cancer care, the completion of therapy presents another phase of cancer care. In this phase, it is important that you understand your risk of recurrence. Though ovarian cancer recurrence depends on the original stage, the surgical outcome, and the response to chemotherapy, recurrences are more the rule than the exception, and recurrence rates in advanced stages range from 50 to 90 percent. Because recurrence is likely, the next phase consists of surveillance, or close observation and monitoring, to assess for cancer recurrence.

This part of survivorship care consists of scheduled follow-up visits with your health care provider, who will evaluate you for signs and symptoms of recurrent ovarian cancer. Most recurrences occur in the first two years after diagnosis, so surveillance visits are more frequent in the beginning. The typical follow-up schedule consists of visits every three months for the first two years, followed by every six months for the next three years. At these visits, your provider will evaluate you for symptoms of recurrent disease. Additionally, you will undergo a complete physical examination. This disease starts in the pelvis, and it is not surprising that most ovarian cancer recurrences occur in the pelvis as well. Therefore, a pelvic examination, including a rectal exam, is an important part of the evaluation. The most commonly experienced signs and symptoms of recurrence are listed in table 13.1. Be sure to talk with your physician about what to do if you develop any symptoms that concern you between visits, so you can be evaluated without delay.

Though different health care providers see patients for follow-up using a similar schedule, there may be some differences among providers in additional testing, based either on provider preferences or on the specific type or stage of cancer. For instance, some ovarian cancers secrete tumor markers, which are detectable by a blood test. If a marker was elevated in your case, testing for this marker may be one way to monitor you for recurrence. Though there are various different tests that may be used, one of the most commonly used tumor markers in ovarian cancer is the CA-125 level. This test is often elevated at the time of diagnosis and can be used to assess the

TABLE 13.1 *Common Signs and Symptoms of Recurrence*

Persistent pain, typically in the abdomen, pelvis, hip, or back
Abdominal bloating or swelling
Feeling a new mass
Vaginal bleeding
Changes in bowel habits
Urinary pressure or frequency
Nausea and/or vomiting
Unexplained weight loss
Cough
Shortness of breath
Worsening fatigue

response to therapy. This number may correlate with disease status and is expected to normalize during or at the completion of primary treatment. This tumor marker can then be followed in the post-treatment period and may be elevated before signs or symptoms of recurrent disease appear. This test is not perfect, however, and may not be elevated in all cases of recurrence. Furthermore, other factors, including infection or inflammation (like diverticulitis), may increase the CA-125 level without other evidence of a recurrence. If a woman is not having symptoms but has an elevated CA-125 test, her care provider may advise a repeat of the test; if an upward trend is noted, further evaluation may be warranted. This number tends to be a major source of anxiety for women who have ovarian cancer; understanding that variations are common can help alleviate anxiety. Talk with your cancer care provider about how tumor markers will be used and interpreted in your surveillance period.

Another part of surveillance that may vary among health care providers is the use of imaging techniques, most often computed axial tomography scans (CT scans, sometimes called CAT scans). A common misconception is that CT scans or other radiographic imaging tests such as magnetic resonance imaging (MRI) or ultrasounds should be done at regular intervals. CT scans are associated with an increased exposure to radiation, which is associated with an increased risk of cancer. Furthermore, studies have shown that when symptoms, examination, and tumor markers are used in combination during the surveillance period, CT scan imaging contributes very little in this period. Though you may undergo CT scan imaging for baseline testing, these scans are often not used for routine surveillance in women who do not have symptoms. Recently, the use of positron emission tomography (PET) with CT scans has become more commonly used in the evaluation of cancer and cancer recurrence. The PET/CT scan is an imaging test that uses a radioactive material to detect areas of increased metabolic activity, which is seen in cancer cells and can help guide management. Currently, CT and PET/CT scans should be reserved for further evaluation of abnormal findings during the physical exam, of symptoms, or of an elevated CA-125 level, and are not recommended for routine surveillance. Of note, if you participate in a clinical trial, you may have specific follow-up testing, including CT scans, that may not be typical of routine follow-up testing. Ask your oncology team about your specific plan for follow-up.

Survivorship Care Plans

After treatment, another important part of the survivorship period is the coordination of care among health care providers—your oncology team and your other doctors. Because you may be receiving your cancer treatment in a hospital other than the hospital where you receive your other care, your treatment and follow-up information is not always readily available for your non-oncology doctors, who may be helping to monitor for cancer recurrence. Unfortunately, non-oncology providers may not be up to date or even comfortable with which tests are needed to provide cancer surveillance, and it is not surprising that a majority of cancer survivors often feel that their doctors do not communicate well. Poor communication can lead to gaps in care, which in turn may result in too little or too much testing, both of which have consequences. Find out what tests you will be receiving and which of your health care providers is taking the lead for your cancer follow-up care.

One way of accomplishing improved communication among providers is to create a survivorship care plan, which may also be referred to as a treatment summary. A survivorship care plan is different from a treatment plan, which is given at the start of treatment and describes the recommended therapies and potential side effects. The survivorship care plan is a document that incorporates the components of cancer diagnosis, treatment, and complications of cancer care. Additionally, the survivorship care plan should include the follow-up schedule and testing that is recommended for surveillance. Though the survivorship care plan is often described during an office visit, it is rarely provided in written form, which means that information gets lost or forgotten. The written survivorship care plan can be created by your oncology team and can then be provided to you and to your other health care providers, so everyone is on the same page.

When communication among providers is optimal, the appropriate testing is performed. Cancer survivors consider communication, including a written survivorship care plan, a priority. Not only does the survivorship care plan enhance communication and coordination among providers, it may also improve patient confidence in the care that is being provided, increase satisfaction, and reduce anxiety for patients and their caregivers.

An example of information that may be incorporated into the survivorship care plan appears in table 13.2. Unfortunately, certain barriers can prevent some providers from creating a survivorship care plan. First, this process can be a time-consuming effort, and office practices are often not equipped with the resources to complete these forms. One solution is to ask for this document in advance, or near the end of treatment. Another option is to take charge of your own information by asking questions, taking notes, and requesting records. Taking charge may empower you and will help you communicate with all your health care providers regarding your care.

TABLE 13.2   *Sample of Information Included in Survivorship Care Plans*

Contact information for oncology and primary care providers
Designation of provider responsible for cancer surveillance
Cancer history
    Cancer stage and type
Surgical procedures performed
    Treatments administered (doses, dates, participation in clinical trials)
    Response to treatment
    Toxicities/side effects experienced
Genetic testing and results (if completed)
Signs and symptoms of cancer recurrence
Possible side effects from treatment and management options
Surveillance recommendations
Routine cancer screening recommendations
Tips for improving health
Support services
    Social work
    Financial counselor
    Community resources

Long-Term and Late Side Effects

Now that treatment has been completed and the follow-up plan has been set, focus should return to finding a sense of well-being. Though it is common to think that now that treatment (chemotherapy) is done, recovery will be quick, patients need to recognize that often late or long-term effects of therapy may continue to affect their daily living. Sometimes these issues appear during treatment and then linger, but often they do not appear until well after treatment has finished. Understanding the differences between treatment side effects and signs of cancer recurrence, though there is some overlap, is critical to getting the best possible care.

We reviewed common symptoms of recurrence earlier. In the following pages we discuss the common late and long-term physical, psychological, and functional effects of treatment in ovarian cancer survivors. These effects can permeate all areas of life.

Physical Effects

Fatigue

One of the most commonly experienced symptoms, both during and after cancer care, is fatigue, or persistent physical or emotional exhaustion related to cancer or cancer treatment. Depending on the severity, fatigue can negatively affect quality of life and can be made worse by other conditions, such as depression, pain, and sleep disturbances. Unfortunately, fatigue is often accepted as an anticipated consequence of cancer care. Checking to make sure that other medical factors, such as anemia and sleep disturbances, are not present should be the first step in addressing fatigue. Medications such as stimulants and psychosocial interventions and counseling have been successful in treating some women's fatigue. Though it may seem counterintuitive, one of the best ways to reduce fatigue is to engage in moderately intense exercise. Exercise recommendations must be made by an expert based on the individual patient's needs and condition.

Pain

Though pain is more often the result of the cancer rather than the treatments, up to 30 percent of cancer survivors continue to experience chronic pain. How best to manage pain depends on the type of symptoms, but options may include physical therapy, medications, acupuncture, or even surgery. Understanding the source of the pain helps guide management. A combination of therapies is often required to relieve pain.

Insomnia

Sleep difficulties, such as difficulty falling or staying asleep, are another common effect of the cancer experience and often result in feelings of fatigue, tiredness, or inability to get things done.

Sleep can be affected by depression or pain, and poor sleep can affect a person's overall well-being. Using medications to aid in sleep or manage pain may be associated with poor sleep quality. Instead, simple improvements in sleep hygiene, such as sleeping at the same time each night, reducing or eliminating television or reading in bed, and avoiding caffeine or sugary foods at night, may help improve the quality of sleep.

Sexual dysfunction

Another significant consequence associated with cancer and its treatment is the development of sexual health issues. Because of the sensitive nature of this topic, patients and providers are both hesitant to discuss it, even though sexual dysfunction affects over 50 percent of gynecologic cancer survivors with problems such as infertility, decreased sexual desire, or pain with intercourse. Some management options include vaginal moisturizers or lubricants and behavioral sexual rehabilitative therapy. Treatment options are tailored to the specific symptoms. Often, both partners must be involved in treatment.

Cognitive deficits (chemo-brain)

Survivors of gynecologic malignancies commonly report that one of the most distressing late effects of treatment are cognitive deficits, which include loss of intellectual function, short-term memory loss, decreased attention span, and lack of concentration. Though it is commonly referred to as chemo-brain, many cancer survivors (and their caregivers) experience these symptoms regardless of the therapies received. This phenomenon can be made worse by fatigue and anxiety, and it certainly may contribute to a lower quality of life. Treatment options include stress management, occupational therapy, neuropsychological evaluation, and stimulant medications. Anticipating changes and keeping your mind stimulated with crossword puzzles, word searches, and reading may help reduce the anxiety associated with these symptoms.

Neuropathy

One of the side effects of chemotherapy, particularly the commonly used platinums and taxanes, is neuropathy, or nerve damage. Symptoms may include ringing in the ears, numbness, and tingling. Numbness or tingling most often occurs in the hands and feet, which may affect daily activities, including walking and balance. If you have numbness in your hands and feet, you need to take safety precautions to minimize injuries from scalds, burns, or falls. Treatment options include antidepressants and antiseizure medications, as well as other options, such as glutathione, vitamin B complex, and acupuncture.

Psychological Distress

Cancer affects not only our physical well-being but also our mental well-being. Unfortunately, a majority of women with gynecologic cancers report some degree of psychological distress. Unlike physical symptoms, which often improve as time passes, psychological distress may last for long periods and affect caregivers and loved ones as well as patients.

Depression

Having cancer is a major life change, which causes feelings of sadness and may bring about or make worse a clinical depression. In addition, physical symptoms such as pain or fatigue may make depression worse—just as depression can make physical symptoms worse. Depression can affect an individual's personal relationships, ability to work effectively, and sense of overall well-being. Having a strong social support system has been shown to reduce the risk of depression. A support system might include family, friends, members of a formal cancer support group (such as those hosted at hospitals), or spiritual or religious groups. Many people benefit from treatment, which might involve counseling, relaxation training, medications, or a combination of therapies.

Anxiety

Another common symptom in cancer survivors and their care-givers is anxiety: anxiety related to worry about financial concerns, physical functioning, general health, or family well-being. Another common cause of anxiety is the fear of cancer recurrence. Many patients have increased anxiety before a visit to their health care provider. Anxiety affects more than 70 percent of cancer survivors. When patients are anxious they may seek more testing than what is needed or recommended, or they may avoid all testing or follow-up visits. The fear of recurrence may be triggered by certain events, such as the anniversary of the surgery date, birthdays, or a new diagnosis of cancer or another illness in a loved one or neighbor. In order to reduce the anxiety associated with the fear of recurrence, we recommend that patients learn the symptoms of cancer recurrence and understand that anxiety will increase around the time of an oncology visit or medical tests associated with cancer evaluation. Support can be provided through psycho-oncology counseling and relaxation training. Strengthening personal relationships, spiritual growth (meditation and practicing gratitude), or participation in support groups may help relieve anxiety and promote well-being.

Functional Effects

Employment

More than 40 percent of cancer survivors are considered to be of working age. The repercussions of cancer can significantly affect work status and performance, and thus can seriously interfere with a person's ability to function. As a cancer survivor, you may have to take long breaks or even leave your job during treatment, but returning to work can be critical in restoring normalcy. When you do return to work, be aware that you may experience difficulties, including cognitive (thinking) or physical limitations. Additionally, factors such as fatigue, depression, and anxiety may also result in the need for specific restrictions, which may continue for years after cancer treatment. Unfortunately, these factors and the limitations that result from them can decrease employment prospects, reduce a person's status at work, or degrade his or her work performance. There may also be real or perceived discrimination by employers or co-workers and decreased job satisfaction.

As a result of cancer and cancer treatment, and all the changes that accompany them, cancer survivors have significantly higher unemployment rates than the general population. It is estimated that more than 50 percent of cancer survivors are unable to work, in some cases because of disabilities from late or long-term effects that not only decrease employment prospects but also contribute to discrimination in hiring. Furthermore, unemployment may result in a loss of health insurance access or affordability, and health insurance is critical for people who have ongoing medical needs.

Financial issues

Clearly, work constraints are often directly related to financial issues, as cancer survivors and their families face increased expenses, both medical and nonmedical costs, such as patient and caregiver days off work, transportation expenses, insurance co-pays, and medical supplies. Furthermore, families affected by cancer are often dealing with decreased income from lost wages, which can create significant financial stressors. The risk of bankruptcy is almost three times higher among people who have cancer than among the general population. There are resources available for financial counseling and assistance programs, including a resource titled *Financial Guidance for Cancer Survivors and Their Families: Off Treatment,* which is available free online at www.cancer.org/acs/groups/content/@editorial/docu ments/document/acsq-020183.pdf or by mail if requested. Other resources include community support groups that may be associated with local cancer awareness as well as support programs or religious establishments.

Improving and Maintaining Healthy Living

After a diagnosis of cancer, it's very worthwhile to spend some time reflecting on how you might improve your health and reduce risk for recurrent disease or the development of new cancers. Not surprisingly, the diagnosis of cancer often serves as a teachable moment, when implementing positive changes are most successful, for both the survivor and her family. Improving general health behaviors has been shown to improve functioning and quality of life. The paragraphs that follow touch on the five primary ways to improve general health: exercise, eat nutritious foods, quit smoking, manage other health conditions, and keep up to date on all recommended cancer screenings.

Exercise

Regular physical activity following cancer treatment can improve recovery after treatment and survival from both cancer and other causes of death. Not only can exercise help reduce cancer risks, but participating in daily activity has been shown to improve fatigue and depression in cancer survivors. The American Cancer Society's recommendations for exercise are available at www.cancer.org. Essentially, the ACS recommends at least 150 minutes of moderate activity each week, which is only 22 minutes a day! Before starting any exercise program, be sure to consult your health care provider to find out if there are any limitations on your physical activities.

Nutrition

Unfortunately, more than two-thirds of the U.S. population is considered overweight, and being overweight is common in cancer survivors just as it is in the rest of the population. Excess weight is associated with increased risk of many different types of cancer, including breast, colon, and endometrial cancers, as well as with other health risks, such as heart disease. Losing even a small amount of weight has been shown to be beneficial to people who are overweight. The American Cancer Society guidelines (available at www.cancer.org) recommend limiting the amount of processed and red meats consumed and eating at least 2.5 cups of vegetables and fruit each day. Choosing whole grains and limiting alcohol intake are also advised. Measuring out your portion sizes will help you control the amount of food you are eating. Cancer survivors, like the rest of the population, do not often follow the American Cancer Society dietary guidelines. But studies in women with breast cancer showed improved survival and well-being with improved nutritional intake, so dietary improvement should be a focus for cancer survivors.

Quit Smoking

Tobacco use directly contributes to the development of a number of cancers and serious medical health problems. Tobacco use is associated with at least 30 percent of all cancer deaths, can increase the complication rates of therapies, and negatively affects survival. Despite these facts, many survivors continue to smoke, which may increase the risk of cancer recurrence or the development of a second malignancy. Though cutting down is a start, cutting down is not good enough. You should not use any tobacco. There are many options to help you quit using tobacco, including self-motivation, smoking cessation classes, nicotine replacements (gum, lozenges, patch), prescription medications (varenicline or bupropion), or integrative medicine with acupuncture or hypnosis. If you smoke, ask your health care provider for additional support.

Managing Other Medical Conditions

Because of risk factors, cancer survivors often have more medical issues than the general population. Though cancer care is often a priority, it is critical that other medical conditions continue to be monitored and managed. As a matter of fact, in patients diagnosed with early-stage cancers, cardiovascular disease, rather than cancer recurrence, is more commonly the cause of death. Yet addressing risk factors for cardiovascular disease is often overlooked, and regrettably, studies have shown that cancer patients receive less care for their other medical problems, particularly heart disease and diabetes, than people who do not have cancer. These gaps in care are further illustrated by a study in which women with ovarian cancer and diabetes were found to have a significantly lower survival rate than their matched nondiabetic counterparts. Therefore, it is as important as ever to ask your primary care providers to discuss risk reduction and management of cardiovascular disease. Because cancer and other medical conditions have a negative effect on one another, coordinating care and promoting ongoing health and treatment of other medical problems is essential.

Routine Cancer Screening

A misconception among cancer survivors is that treatment for one cancer prevents other cancers as well. However, the opposite is actually true: cancer survivors remain at high risk for secondary cancers due to common risk factors and treatment complications. For instance, certain chemotherapy agents can increase the risk for leukemia, and tamoxifen therapy for breast cancer can increase the risk of endometrial cancer. Therefore, in addition to being evaluated for recurrence, cancer survivors should continue with all recommended cancer screening. This includes standard evaluations with mammograms for breast cancer detection; colonoscopy for colorectal cancers; and if appropriate, Pap and human papillomavirus (HPV) testing for cervical cancers. Ask your primary care and oncology providers about symptoms to be on the lookout for and what other tests you will need for cancer prevention and early detection.

Conclusion

The completion of therapy is a huge milestone and leads into another phase of cancer care. In this chapter we've emphasized why it's important for you to discuss the follow-up plans and tests with your cancer provider, and to understand and adhere to those plans. Doing so can reduce anxiety and can improve the coordination of cancer care. Dealing with the aftereffects of cancer and its treatment is a central focus of survivorship care. Taking care of yourself for healthy living is necessary to help get you back to the best state of health. And because it is the family that gets cancer, including your support system in this process can be invaluable.

Though cancer is a life-changing experience, we hope you can find the opportunity to use it as a positive chance for growth. This philosophy, which is also known as post-traumatic growth, can increase your sense of strength and improve relationships with friends and family. As the number of women living with ovarian cancer or a history of ovarian cancer increases, the understanding of survivorship care will continue to improve and allow for a better transition to wellness.

A Personal Perspective on Coping with Recurrences, Maintaining Hope, and Connecting with the Survivor Community

Annie Ellis

I was diagnosed with ovarian cancer in 2004 at the age of 40. I had no risk fac-tors—I am Filipina and Puerto Rican with a very low incidence of cancer in a very large extended family. The first four years were pretty rough, with two recurrences, three major surgeries, five chemotherapy regimens, and a remission vaccine clini-cal trial. I am currently enjoying an unexpected very long third remission.

My first remission was filled with anxiety. Life felt like a minefield as I tried to do and eat all the "right" things. There's an overwhelming amount of information on the Internet, and news headlines don't tell the whole story. I spent a lot of time at support groups and was introduced to trusted resources for information. For me, my first recurrence was harder than the original diagnosis. I found hope by meeting recurrent survivors and learned that there are different ways to cope, survive, and thrive. I attended survivor courses and conferences and heard about the many exciting drugs in development and the strategy of using clinical trials to expand our treatment options.

Things got really tough during my second recurrence. A standard chemo-therapy kept things stable for a while and then stopped working. I had lots of time to think while seeking three second opinions to explore my options. Was this now a chronic condition? How much time did I have left? And what did I want to do with that time? I also thought about the worst-case scenario. My mind went to some very dark places, but I found that I could still have hope about what I would want the end of my journey to look like. I know I want to remain active for as long as possible, be free from pain, and continue to be me. I found hope by talking to survivors who were living with chronic disease and living well—remaining active, traveling, maintaining a sense of humor, and finding something to enjoy every day! Meeting others managing disease long term showed me that I, too, could find a way to live with chronic ovarian cancer if it ever came to that.

Connecting with other survivors and learning more about this disease has helped me improve communications with my medical team. Knowing what's important to me helped me have clear discussions about my goals and what side effects I am willing to tolerate. Do I want to attend a special function or travel? Do I hope to keep my hair or avoid neuropathy? Sometimes other options are possible, and sometimes they are not, but we don't know unless we ask. I have also become better at reporting side effects to my medical team and in asking for help with things that affect daily living, like sleep issues, pain, depression, and sexuality.

This third remission has lasted longer than anyone expected and I have had amazing opportunities to serve the ovarian cancer community as a research advocate, as well as share the hope with other survivors. I don't know what the future holds, but no matter what happens, I am not alone.

CHAPTER 14

Managing Recurrent Disease

Leslie M. Randall, MD

A fter treatment for ovarian cancer, most women will be *in re-mission*. This means that there is no evidence of measurable cancer according to a thorough physical examination, CA-125 (and/or HE4) blood testing, and, at times, radiographic imaging. Being in re-mission is also referred to as being *disease-free* or as having *no evidence of disease* (NED). After treatment, patients are monitored every three to six months by an oncologist who reviews any symptoms, performs a physical examination, and checks CA-125 blood test results. If any of these parameters is not in the normal range, there is concern that the cancer has regrown. Oncologists call tumor regrowth *recurrent disease.*

Recurrence of disease is a very unwelcome event for women, their families, and their medical team. Making matters worse is that about 75 percent of women who are diagnosed with Stage III or IV ovarian cancer will experience recurrent disease. Most women with a history of ovarian cancer who experience recurrent disease will have options for further treatment, in contrast to many other types of cancer that have few options to treat cancer recurrence. Therefore, managing re-current disease is something that many gynecologic oncologists and their ovarian cancer patients spend a majority of their time doing.

Likewise, an intense international research effort is devoted to finding safe and effective solutions to recurrent ovarian cancer.

What Happens if I Get Recurrent Disease?

The sad truth that frustrates patients and doctors alike is that most women who experience a recurrence of their ovarian cancer cannot be cured. While this news can devastate the heart and spirit, it is important to know that in many cases, all hope is not lost. Even though recurrent ovarian cancer is technically not curable, many patients can remain alive and functional for quite some time after this diagnosis. Understandably, most women, maybe because they are the consummate planners and managers, would prefer to know how long "quite some time" really is. Unfortunately, no doctor is able to reliably predict the length of time a woman will survive after she has been diagnosed with recurrent ovarian cancer. That being said, some particulars of a woman's general health and ovarian cancer status can provide a ballpark measure of prognosis. Doctors refer to these particulars as *prognostic factors*. Prognostic factors can also predict what treatments are likely to work against the cancer and what treatments are likely not to work. These prognostic factors, listed in table 14.1, provide categories of recurrent ovarian cancer that can guide treatment recommendations.

How Is Recurrent Disease Diagnosed?

Most cancer recurrences are diagnosed when women who are in remission from ovarian cancer develop new symptoms, such as bloat-

TABLE 14.1 *Prognostic Factors for Ovarian Cancer*

- Age (younger is better)
- Performance status (a measure of physical activity; more active is better)
- Success of the first operation (optimal versus suboptimal)
- Time passed between the last platinum chemotherapy and the diagnosis of recurrence (longer is better; at least 6 months defines platinum sensitivity)
- BRCA gene mutation status (BRCA mutation carriers generally live longer than noncarriers)

---

ing or localized pain; have new abnormal findings on their physical examination; or experience an increase in their CA-125 level during their follow-up time. For many women, two or three of these events will happen at the same time. Sometimes recurrent disease is suspected only because the CA-125 blood test is slowly rising, but there are no other signs or symptoms of cancer. In these cases, the elevated CA-125 must be confirmed by showing a consistent rise over time. Measuring changes in CA-125 values requires drawing more than one blood test over a specified period, usually at least one month, depending on how high the CA-125 value is. For example, high values (CA-125 >100) are more suspicious for recurrent disease than low levels and can be confirmed quickly. If the CA-125 level is lower than 100, it can take longer to identify a definite pattern. There is no specific CA-125 level that is diagnostic of recurrence; however, a significant increase (for example a doubling) from an individual patient's baseline level (generally the stable range of lowest values once in remission) is suspicious for disease recurrence. At times, CA-125 levels can rise for reasons that are completely unrelated to the cancer, such as inflammation and other illnesses. If the CA-125 test continues to rise, recurrence is suspected. This suspicion needs to be confirmed with some form of imaging, exam, or biopsy. There is no *standard of care* to help the oncologist diagnose recurrent disease, and every case is different in terms of which of these tests needs to be or will be done to confirm the diagnosis of cancer recurrence.

How Is Recurrent Disease Managed?

Doctors and researchers are still discovering and learning the nuances of managing recurrent ovarian cancer. Every case is different. Every woman is different. Multiple factors determine the treatment recommendation for each individual patient, some of which are patient-dependent, like general health and nutrition status. Factors related to the cancer are also important, such as the number of and location of the recurrent tumors. There are myriad options, and at least at this time, no right answer regarding which treatment is best. In general, the primary treatment is more chemotherapy, though some women will be candidates for more surgery, and fewer will be candidates for radiation.

There are now several laboratory tests designed to predict which chemotherapy treatments will or will not work for an individual patient. Each test is a little different. Some treat a sample of an individual tumor in the test tube (*in vitro*) with various chemotherapies to see which will work best. This is similar to how researchers test infections in a culture and antibiotic-sensitivity test. Although it was expected that the chemotherapy-sensitivity tests would be as good as antibiotic assays, these tests have not been as accurate as hoped. The main problem is with the treatments themselves, not the test. Until more effective treatments for ovarian cancer are developed, the in vitro tests will remain of limited value. Luckily, this situation is changing for the better. We are starting to get some more specific clues about how individual types of ovarian cancer differ and how they can be better treated. Many new types of treatment are being developed that help the body's own immune system fight off cancer or attack the tumor machinery in a more specific way than traditional chemotherapy does. In addition, the biological factors in the patient, called *biomarkers,* which predict the effectiveness of the new therapy in the individual, are more advanced now than ever. Until these new treatments are "ready for prime time," oncologists rely on the prognostic factors listed in table 14.1 to recommend options for follow-up treatment.

When deciding how to treat recurrent ovarian cancer, the first thing to consider is what oncologists call the *platinum-free interval.* This is the time that has passed between the last dose of platinum-based chemotherapy and the diagnosis of the recurrence. This interval is an important factor used to determine the following:

- if a woman is a candidate for another surgery
- how well the cancer will likely respond to chemotherapy retreatment
- how severe the side effects of surgery or subsequent chemotherapy will be
- a woman's long-term outlook, or prognosis

When more than six months have passed since the last platinum-based chemotherapy, women are classified as having a *platinum-sensitive* recurrence. In general, women with platinum-sensitive recurrence are retreated with platinum-based chemotherapy, are considered potential candidates for repeated surgery, and have a better prognosis for longevity. Conversely, when fewer than six months have passed, women are classified as having *platinum-resistant* recurrence. In general, platinum-resistant cancer is less responsive to repeated chemotherapy treatments than its platinum-sensitive counterpart. Therefore, these women are typically treated with non-platinum-containing chemotherapy, and the risks of surgery often outweigh any benefits for them. Some oncologists consider a patient whose cancer recurs between six and twelve months since the last chemotherapy to be *intermediately* platinum sensitive. This group poses somewhat of a dilemma in terms of what treatment will be best and whether surgery is advisable. Over the long term, women in this category will "declare themselves" as either platinum sensitive or platinum resistant—meaning it will become clear whether platinum chemotherapy is effective for them.

If the cancer grows during the first chemotherapy course, women are classified as having *platinum-refractory* cancer. These cancers can be very aggressive and are often not responsive to chemotherapy. Cancer often grows during chemotherapy treatment for recurrent disease, but this is not considered to be as bad for prognosis as when the cancer gets worse on the first chemotherapy. Platinum sensitivity is not all black and white, however. In reality platinum sensitivity exists on a scale. In other words, there are gray zones in which the patient and oncologist work together to decide which treatment is the best choice in the given situation.

Platinum-Sensitive Recurrence

Surgery

Women with platinum-sensitive recurrence of ovarian cancer are considered to be potential candidates for another cytoreductive surgery. The decision to do surgery for recurrent ovarian cancer is complicated for both the surgeon and the patient. In most cases, minimally invasive surgery is not a good option in this situation. Therefore, these surgeries must be performed under general anesthesia through a large vertical incision in the middle of the abdomen, similar to that required for the first surgery. This makes the risk-benefit balance controversial, and we currently don't have good quality medical data to define the risk-benefit balance. The controversy stems from two main concerns about surgery. First is the lack of randomized, prospective evidence that repeated surgery is helpful to fight the cancer. There is, however, an increasing body of retrospective research indicating that successful surgery (resection of all gross disease) in appropriately selected patients (good performance status, three or fewer sites of recurrence, platinum-sensitive disease) is associated with longer survival. Second is the risk of serious surgical complications and chemotherapy delays in women who undergo second (or third, or fourth) surgeries. Two large clinical trials are under way to give more information on how helpful surgery is for women with recurrent cancer. In the meantime, surgeons use their knowledge of the cancer and its behavior, the patient's general health, and the patient's preferences to decide whether to proceed with repeated surgery prior to restarting chemotherapy.

The rationale supporting repeated surgery is similar to the rationale for recommending the first surgery—to reduce the amount of cancer the chemotherapy has to treat and to alleviate disease symptoms. Most surgeons would agree that surgery is probably helpful for the properly selected patient. Patient selection is a judgment call that is guided by a lot of training and experience. Our current best judgment with regard to who is a "good" candidate for repeated surgery can be found in table 14.2, but the main important factors are whether the patient has a platinum-sensitive recurrence and whether all the cancer can be safely removed. Although any platinum-sensitive patient can be considered for repeat surgery, those with very long platinum-free intervals (one year or more) are the best candidates. Likewise, those who have few tumors in areas safe for removal are also the best candidates. Just like the initial surgery, the goal is to remove all visible cancer. Studies are showing that this is even more important in repeat surgery than in the first surgery. Currently, surgeons use CT scans and physical exams to decide whose

- Age
- Performance status
- Platinum sensitivity (the longer the better)
- Recurrent cancer limited to 3 or fewer tumors
- Absence of abdominal fluid (ascites)
- Tumor location in areas safe for removal
- Likely removal of all cancer

tumors can probably be completely removed. In most cases, however, it is impossible to know whether all tumors can be removed with any certainty without doing the surgery. Some doctors perform a less invasive look into the abdomen through a small incision (laparoscopy) for diagnostic purposes before proceeding with the attempt at the bigger repeat surgery.

The main argument against repeat surgery is that its risks cannot be justified in a cancer that, technically, cannot be cured. Most women will have a full recovery from surgery, but the complication risks for a repeat surgery are relatively high. This is because women have scar tissue from the first surgery and lingering effects from any previous chemotherapy, and they can be nutritionally depleted and not in the best physical condition for surgery to begin with. Add to this a sometimes technically challenging and long operation on cancerous tumors and scar tissue, and then follow that with chemotherapy again. It quickly becomes clear why repeated surgeries can be risky. Some women might be candidates for surgery through small incisions for a less invasive procedure, but even a small-incision, or laparoscopic, procedure being done to remove recurrent cancer carries significant risks. The next few sections will detail potential complications from surgery.

Incision complications

The surgery is usually performed through a long vertical incision in the abdomen. Most women who are candidates for surgery have already had at least one prior abdominal procedure with the same type of incision. This incision causes short-term pain and disability, both of which can be treated with medication and minor rehabilitation. Incisions can become infected (*abscess*), collect fluid (*seroma*), or bleed (*hematoma*), and they can even come apart or open. A wound that doesn't stay closed is called a *dehiscence*. Dehiscence is an inconvenient cosmetic problem if it happens at the skin level. Skin dehiscence is usually treated with a wound packing or suction sponge and allowed to heal "from the inside out." This is called *secondary intention* and can take days to weeks depending on how deep the incision is. Overweight women have a higher risk for dehiscence and all other wound complications, and it takes them longer to heal from a given problem than it does women with normal weight.

In extreme cases, dehiscence occurs on the level of the *fascia*, a strong connective tissue that holds the entire abdomen together and keeps the intestines inside. Dehiscence of the fascia can be a dramatic and frightening experience for the patient. Surgeons view fascial dehiscence as a life-threatening emergency that requires immediate return to the operating room for repair.

Hemorrhage

Just as for the first surgery, bleeding and hemorrhage are major risks for the second surgery. Scar tissue from the first surgery distorts the normal anatomy, making bleeding harder to avoid the second or third time around. Also, prior chemotherapy interferes with the body's ability to stop bleeding. The amount and type of prior chemotherapy, in addition to the time elapsed since the last dose, determines whether chemotherapy will make the bleeding risk higher.

Gynecologic oncology surgeons are well trained to avoid and treat excessive bleeding. Numerous techniques aid the surgeon's judgment and skill when it comes to blood loss. The technique with the most potential long-term consequences for patients is blood transfusion. Transfusion of donated blood products can be life saving, but it is prohibited by some religions and carries a small risk of transmitting infections like HIV and hepatitis B or C. While the risk of infection is real, it is also very small, thanks to universal and accurate testing of donated blood for these infections. The more likely complication to have with blood transfusion is an allergic reaction to another person's blood. Allergic reactions to blood happen when a patient has developed antibodies or immunity to antigens in another person's blood after receiving a previous transfusion. Thus, the reaction is more likely to happen if the patient has received blood transfusions in the past, and past transfusions are not uncommon among ovarian cancer patients who have had previous surgery and chemotherapy.

Infection

Patients with recurrent cancer who have repeat surgeries are at risk for serious infections. Most infections are a result of the surgery itself, usually involving incisions in the skin, the intestine, or the vagina. These infections are treated with a combination of antibiotics and needle drainage procedures, but sometimes a return to the operating room is needed to repair the infection surgically. Some women will experience a *nosocomial* infection, an infection contracted in the hospital from other patients. Nosocomial infections include pneumonia, *Clostridium difficile* (*C. diff*) diarrhea, and methicillin-resistant staphylococcus aureus (MRSA) of the skin. Repeat surgery patients are at a particularly high risk for nosocomial infections because they typically have relatively long hospital stays following the long and complex surgery. In addition, previous chemotherapy and the cancer itself increase the risk of these infections.

Intestinal injury

Previous extensive surgeries like cytoreductive procedures create scar tissue (adhesions) around the internal organs and change the way the organs are placed within the abdomen. Performing surgery is similar to trying to find your way to a familiar location but needing to drive there via many detours. Operating in this rerouted environment is challenging. Gynecologic oncologists are specially trained to work through these adhesions without damaging any of the internal organs, but sometimes injuries are unavoidable. As with any other complication of surgery, this complication can happen even with the best of surgeons. Luckily, these injuries are usually noticed and can be fixed right away, but fixing an injury might require removing that portion of the intestine or a permanent colostomy (in a colostomy, the large intestine is diverted to drain from the skin on the abdomen into a bag called an *appliance*). If bowel injuries are not recognized at the time of surgery, or if they are incompletely repaired, a life-threatening situation can occur. Though this complication is not common, it is also not rare, and complications such as these interfere with the patient's ability to get timely chemotherapy.

Delay of chemotherapy

Chemotherapy is the essential treatment for recurrent ovarian cancer. Even though taking time to heal from surgery before starting chemotherapy sounds like a great idea, a long delay (more than three weeks) can allow the cancer to regrow following the surgery. If the cancer regrows before the chemotherapy is restarted, some of the benefit from surgery is lost. Therefore, if surgery is possible but likely to result in a long recovery, the surgeon might advise against it. These decisions are guided by the surgeon's judgment and experience. Predicting exactly how long a delay the surgery will cause is not possible.

Chemotherapy

Chemotherapy is essential for treatment of ovarian cancer recurrence, and unlike with most other cancers, many chemotherapy regimens are available for women faced with this diagnosis. Unlike the first time around, there is not a set or standard number of times (cycles) the chemotherapy will need to be given to control the cancer. Some women will go back into remission after six to eight rounds of treatment, just like the first time around. It is not uncommon, however, for a woman to need to have more than eight rounds of chemotherapy for recurrence. Again, the most important factor to determine which regimen is recommended is the platinum-free interval. The platinum-free interval predicts which treatment will work best. Also important to consider are any lingering side effects from the previous chemotherapy. The usual recommended chemotherapy for platinum-sensitive patients is a two-drug regimen that includes carboplatin. We often call this a *platinum doublet*.

Clinical trials have established three main platinum doublets as the go-to treatments for platinum-sensitive recurrence. These doublets combine the carboplatin with either paclitaxel, as given for the first chemotherapy, Doxil (pegylated liposomal doxorubicin, or PLD), or Gemzar (gemcitabine). These three options are considered roughly equivalent, but only carboplatin/paclitaxel and carboplatin/PLD have been compared in a head-to-head trial. The clinical trial that led to FDA approval of carboplatin/Gemzar compared the activity of the doublet to carboplatin by itself, but carboplatin/Gemzar has not been compared to the other two doublets. A popular variation of the carboplatin/Gemzar doublet is to substitute cisplatin for carboplatin because there is an important synergy between cisplatin and Gemzar. Whether this substitution makes a difference has not been studied in a clinical trial.

If these different combinations are roughly equivalent, how does the doctor choose which one to recommend? Because the different doublets have roughly the same effectiveness against the cancer, the decision regarding which one is best can focus on what side effect profile and chemotherapy schedule is most desirable to the patient.

Choosing Based on Side Effects

Since all these regimens include carboplatin, they will all have the common side effects of nausea and lowered counts of blood cells that fight anemia (red cells and hemoglobin), infection (white cells), and bleeding (platelets). In addition, women getting carboplatin a second time around (or more) can have an allergic reaction to the drug. This is a serious, potentially life-threatening side effect that infusion center staff are trained to treat quickly. The second drug in the doublet, however, dictates how the side effects will be different among the three options.

Paclitaxel tends to be the first choice for recurrence, but it has two main side effects that most women would prefer to avoid: hair loss and peripheral neuropathy (numbness, pain, or tingling in the hands and feet). Some women may have neuropathy from previous use of paclitaxel that might even interfere with daily activities. If this is the case, the neuropathy will likely get worse if paclitaxel is given again. In cases where the doctor determines that the neuropathy is at a critically high level, paclitaxel should be avoided because worsening neuropathy can have an irreversible and very negative effect on the ability to walk, write, sew, play an instrument, or perform other tasks. It is questionable whether it's a good idea to subject women to this poor quality of life when the treatment will likely not be curative. If the treatment were able to cure the cancer, then these risks might be more justified. This does not mean that paclitaxel should never be used. Paclitaxel can be very effective for recurrent cancer. The best strategy is to give paclitaxel only to women who have no or mild neuropathy to start with and then monitor them frequently for worsening. If the neuropathy gets worse, the paclitaxel should then be stopped. Other taxanes, like docetaxel or nab-paclitaxel (Abraxane), can be substituted for paclitaxel and bring about less neuropathy in some cases.

The carboplatin/PLD doublet has become popular among women because it is effective and has a more favorable side effect profile than the carboplatin/paclitaxel doublet. Women on carboplatin/PLD do not experience hair loss, so the wigs and scarves can stay in the closet. They are also not at risk for worsening neuropathy, which is especially helpful if the patient has moderate to severe neuropathy from the previous chemotherapy treatments. An additional benefit is that carboplatin/PLD is given on an every-28-day cycle, providing women with more time off to enjoy life between doses.

The carboplatin/PLD doublet does carry the extra risk of a rash on the palms and soles of the feet called *palmar-* (for hand) *plantar-* (for feet) *erythro-* (for red) *dysesthesia* (for pain), or PPE for short. This painful red rash is thought to happen because the PLD can be excreted in the sweat and then get trapped by heat and pressure from the shoes or hand friction. PPE has also been reported in waistband and bra strap areas. This rash is generally managed best by prevention—keeping the hands and feet cool and well ventilated while on the PLD drug. A good rule of thumb is to treat the feet like the feet of a person who has diabetes, and wear loose-fitting, comfortable shoes. The worst PPE I have seen in my practice has been with women wearing flip-flops and sandals. My patients who wear cotton socks and well-fitted casual shoes do much better. It is also good to rotate pairs of shoes to avoid repetitive pressure on one area or another.

A recent challenge with giving carboplatin/PLD has been a PLD shortage in the United States. The drug's only manufacturer had to stop production, leaving the United States without a supply for nearly two years. When manufacture started again, it was in limited quantities. After an executive order from President Barack Obama, the FDA facilitated the import of a nearly identical version of PLD from an overseas manufacturer. The U.S. manufacturer has now restored production, but the supply is still considered vulnerable to future shortages.

A third option for women with platinum-sensitive recurrent ovarian cancer is the carboplatin/Gemzar doublet. This regimen is given on a day 1 and day 8 schedule every 21 days. It is the most time-intensive of the three options. The main side effects of carboplatin/Gemzar are related to lowered blood cell counts, especially the platelets that counteract excessive bleeding. Unlike booster shots for white blood cells and iron or transfusion for anemia, there is no good antidote for drops in the platelet count. The best management of this change in red blood cell counts (called *thrombocytopenia*) is to reduce the dose of the chemotherapy. Dose reductions have the potential to reduce the ability of the chemotherapy to fight the cancer but are probably not an issue unless the dose has to be dramatically lowered from the prescribed dose.

Women who have platinum-sensitive recurrence but are not in good physical condition can still be helped by chemotherapy with carboplatin by itself, to avoid the side effects of the combined drugs.

Maintenance

Most women will need at least six to eight rounds of the chosen chemotherapy to get into remission. Building on the "recurrent treatment is helpful but not a cure" theme, we have studied a strategy to continue low-dose treatment for up to one year after chemotherapy is done, in an attempt to keep cancer away as long as possible. The best treatment to give as a maintenance strategy is one that is more convenient, with fewer side effects, than standard chemotherapy. The most successful maintenance treatments in clinical trials to date have been with Avastin, or bevacizumab, and olaparib.

Avastin is a "new" type of chemotherapy treatment in that it does not attack rapidly growing cells in the body such as cancer, the gut, and hair follicles. Rather, it disables a protein in the blood that helps cancerous tumors steal blood vessels, oxygen, and nutrients from the patient's body to fuel the growth of the cancer. The advantage of this *biologic* type of treatment is that there are different side effects than with standard chemotherapy. Therefore, women on Avastin get a break from the fatigue, hair loss, neuropathy, and bone marrow suppression that come with standard treatment but are still able to fight the cancer. Unfortunately, there are still risks when Avastin is used. The side effects of Avastin are mostly related to the drug's effect on blood vessels and include high blood pressure, kidney proteins in the urine (called *proteinuria*), nosebleeds, and headaches. These side effects are usually mild to moderate and can be treated with increased monitoring and blood pressure medications.

Some side effects of this drug, however, are severe and life threatening. These severe adverse events include heart attack, stroke, blood clots, and bowel perforation (a hole in the intestine). These side effects are so bad you would think Avastin would be pulled from the market, but the reality is that these severe effects are very rare—rare enough that less than 5 percent of women on Avastin experience these effects. The benefits of Avastin in fighting the cancer typically outweigh this risk. Some women are at a particularly high risk for these side effects, say, if they have uncontrolled high blood pressure or problems with their intestines like a blockage or inflammation, and will not be considered good candidates for this treatment. As always, the risks of the treatment need to be weighed against the benefits. In clinical trials, maintenance Avastin has delayed the time to recurrence but has not resulted in more cures or longer overall lifespan. Therefore, this risk-and-benefit tug-of-war has prevented Avastin from receiving FDA approval at this time. Women may still be able to receive Avastin treatment if their physician recommends it; however, some insurance companies may not agree to pay for it without approval from the FDA.

Olaparib inhibits a protein that allows the cells to repair DNA damage caused by chemotherapy. It might also work to directly kill cancer cells. Olaparib works best in women who are known carriers of the BRCA1 or BRCA2 gene mutation, but it can work for women with platinum-sensitive recurrences who are not known BRCA gene-mutation carriers. In December 2014, the FDA approved olaparib (Lynparza) for treatment of recurrent ovarian cancer in women with known BRCA1 or BRCA2 mutations and who have been treated with three or more previous chemotherapy regimens. More study is required before olaparib can be considered for FDA approval in other clinical situations.

Platinum-Resistant Recurrence

Platinum-resistant ovarian cancer is defined as cancer that recurs within six months of finishing the last dose of chemotherapy received. Some clinicians and researchers consider those who experience cancer recurrence within twelve months of the last chemotherapy to also be platinum-resistant. Treating platinum-resistant cancer is very challenging. There are several options for the treatment of platinum-resistant disease, but none of them has a great track record for inducing long-term remission. This fact leads to an important principle of treatment planning: surgery, in general, is not a good option for these women, because the chemotherapy required to help the surgery fight the cancer is often not very effective for them. This shifts the risk-benefit balance toward risk and away from benefit, but there are exceptions to this rule. Some women will need surgery because the cancer is blocking a certain part of the intestines or the urinary system. Also, if the patient has never had a *maximal effort* cytoreductive surgery performed by a gynecologic oncologist (i.e., a dedicated attempt to remove all disease by a qualified surgeon), the previous less-than-maximal surgery might explain the short duration of chemotherapy effect. Therefore, surgery might be recommended at this time for these women.

Because chemotherapy is not as effective as we would like, many oncologists consider new cancer treatments that are only available on clinical trials as the first choice for treatment of women with platinum-resistant cancer. However, finding a clinical trial can be challenging. Even oncologists who work on clinical trials are not always aware of all studies available to patients. In the United States, all clinical trials in progress are required to be registered on the website www.clinicaltrials.gov. This site has a search engine where the patient can type in "ovarian cancer" and her geographic location. These searches often produce an overwhelming number of results, many of which will be irrelevant to the person's specific situation. Here, it's important to enlist the help of your oncologist to look at each opportunity. Unfortunately, doctors' schedules do not easily accommodate this time-consuming job, but most will help in the search for appropriate clinical trials in the best interest of their patients.

If a clinical trial is not available or desired, some fairly standard options for treatment were established by previous clinical trials. These include the previously mentioned doublets but without the carboplatin: single-agent PLD, paclitaxel, Gemzar, or Avastin. Other options include a drug called topotecan or treatment with a drug called cyclophosphamide. The National Comprehensive Cancer Network (NCCN) has a compendium list of drugs acceptable for use in recurrent ovarian cancer; these are listed in table 14.3.

TABLE 14.3   *Chemotherapy Drugs Used to Treat Recurrent Disease*

Platinum-sensitive recurrence	Carboplatin/paclitaxel (or docetaxel)
	Carboplatin/pegylated liposomal doxorubicin (PLD)
	Carboplatin (or cisplatin)/gemcitabine
	Carboplatin or cisplatin alone
Platinum-resistant recurrence	Investigational new drug on clinical trial
	PLD (+/– Avastin)
	Bevacizumab
	Topotecan (+/– Avastin)
	Weekly paclitaxel (+/– Avastin)
	Docetaxel
	Nab-paclitaxel
	Etoposide (oral)
Other acceptable single agents	altretamine
	capecitabine
	cyclophosphamide
	doxorubicin
	ifosfamide
	irinotecan
	melphalan
	pemetrexed
	vinorelbine

SOURCE: National Comprehensive Cancer Network.

Platinum Refractory

Women who have cancer that gets worse while on their first chemotherapy are in a very difficult situation. Currently, no treatment options are particularly beneficial. Like patients who are platinum resistant, these patients are best served by participating in a clinical trial that is testing a new drug. Unfortunately, many trials exclude platinum-refractory patients because the cancer is affecting their general health, making it less safe to give them experimental drugs. Contrary to what is depicted on television, oncologists are overly cautious, not overly incautious, when testing new treatments. Their attitude reflects their concern for patient welfare.

What if Another Remission Doesn't Happen?

If a patient does not go into remission on a given chemotherapy regimen, either a new treatment is recommended or, if the patient is tolerating the therapy well, the current treatment can be continued until the cancer starts to grow back and is no longer responding to that therapy.

Radiation Therapy

Radiation therapy can be very effective to control symptoms from tumors that are not removable with surgery. It is generally reserved for tumors that are limited to one area and that are causing symptoms. The side effects of radiation depend on the area that is treated and can be short term or long term. Short-term effects by definition resolve after the treatment is over, but long-term effects—like abnormal connections, called *fistulae*, between the bowels and vagina or skin that result in bowel contents leaking out of these areas—can be life changing. A decision about whether to do radiation depends on the likely side effects and the area that needs to be treated.

Palliative Care

Palliative care is a philosophy and a practice in medicine whose priority is managing symptoms that patients experience as a result of their cancer and its treatment. Sometimes oncologists provide palliative care to their patients, but many centers now have specialists with extra training and certification in palliative care. Unfortunately, palliative care is often confused with hospice and end-of-life care. Many doctors will not recommend palliative care, and many women will refuse it, because of their false perception that accepting palliative care means "giving up" on the cancer patient, or relegating the patient to a "death sentence." These phrases, unfortunately, are frequently heard when palliative care is being discussed.

Palliative care is very underused in ovarian cancer care. It is usually started late in the course of cancer treatment, when there is not enough time left for women to get the most out of its many benefits. Contrary to common perception, women can receive cancer treatments and be enrolled in palliative care at the same time. There are palliative care companies that provide in-home nursing visits to help educate patients and their families and prevent emergency room visits and hospital admissions. In the oncology world, there is a new conversation about using early palliative care to improve disease, treatment education and quality of life, and even prolong survival time for patients battling cancer. Because women can live a relatively long time with ovarian cancer, palliative care is all the more important to help women with the side effects from cancer and treatment that add up over time.

Some conditions caused by the cancer are particularly challenging to ovarian cancer patients, causing obstruction or dysfunction of the digestive (intestinal) system, fluid in the abdomen (ascites), fluid on the lungs (pleural effusion), and poorly controlled pain. These symptoms must be aggressively managed with palliative measures to preserve quality of life.

Malignant bowel obstruction is a condition where a cancer tumor either physically blocks the intestine or causes a paralysis that significantly slows down the movement of food through the digestive system. Determining which problem is causing the symptoms is essential to providing the patient with the best treatment. Regardless of the cause, however, the first step in helping patients is to temporarily stop intake of food or drink by mouth, allowing the intestines to rest. This "bowel rest" often allows the bowels to "reset" and start working better. Sometimes a suction tube that drains the stomach and is inserted through the nose can help as well. Though the insertion of this suction tube is uncomfortable for the patient, stomach drainage through the tube often gives the patient a great deal of relief.

If the obstruction is complete blockage, surgery is often recommended. If surgery is performed, there are a few ways to relieve the blockage. To understand these options, it might help to envision the intestinal blockage as a knot tied in a garden hose that is blocking the flow of water. The most desirable surgical option is to remove the section of intestine with the knot, or blockage, and reconnect the two ends of the bowel internally. If this is not possible, then sometimes the bowel can be routed around the blockage. This surgery is called *diversion*. Diversions can be from one part of the intestine to another, or from the intestine to the skin surface by a colostomy, or a bag. Colostomies done for recurrent cancer are more often permanent than not. Any time surgery is performed for intestinal blockage, the risk for complications and for a new obstruction down the road is high.

The more common condition blocking the intestine is called *carcinomatous ileus. Ileus* is an intestinal paralysis, and *carcinomatous* means that it is caused by extensive covering of the intestine with hundreds of tiny tumors that interfere with the muscle contractions that move food through the digestive tract. Because carcinomatous ileus involves large portions of the bowel, surgical repair is not effective. Chemotherapy and diet changes are the best treatment. Important principles of dietary change are to eat small, frequent meals with high calories, proteins, vitamins, and minerals. Nutrition shakes and baby food are helpful. Bulky fiber and high volumes of liquids are usually not tolerated.

Ascites, or fluid in the abdomen, caused by the cancer can be a very uncomfortable problem that is best alleviated by chemotherapy. When chemotherapy is not working, the fluid can be drained with a needle in the skin. Drainage usually provides tremendous short-term relief, but if the cancer is not treatable with chemotherapy, the fluid will quickly return after the drainage—within two or three days. If women are candidates for more chemotherapy, small and repeated drainage procedures can be done. If women are not candidates for more chemotherapy, then a permanent catheter can be placed to drain the fluid any time the patient has discomfort from the pressure. Any drainage procedure will deplete the body of hydration and proteins. Most women with ascites are also having difficulty eating and drinking. Therefore it can be almost impossible for them to get rehydrated and replace the protein with their diet alone. This makes women unstable for continued chemotherapy, so the drainage needs to be done with caution and with the long-term plan in mind.

This chapter has reviewed the relevant terminology and diagnostic methods surrounding the diagnosis of ovarian cancer recurrence. It has also covered many of the more common treatment options and palliative care interventions that are available today. Ultimately, the management of disease recurrence in a woman who has ovarian cancer is most successful when it is individualized based on the woman's health status, disease characteristics, and life goals.

A Personal Perspective on Considering the End of Life

Bev Lipsitz

I've been living with Stage IV ovarian cancer for over five years. During that time I've attended a monthly support group and a summer weekend retreat, both for women with ovarian cancer, so I've come to know many other women in my situation.

There are a few women I think of as the lucky few, women whose cancer has never recurred. But most of the women I've known have had one or more recurrences.

Many of these women go in and out of treatment over the first few months or years. The treatment works, and for a while the cancer goes into hiding (official status: no evidence of disease; affectionately: dancing with NED).

Life is good until the next recurrence, and the cycle begins again.

In most cases, each cycle from recurrence to treatment to recurrence is shorter than the last, until the best that can be hoped for is "stable disease," when treatment can delay progression but never bring back NED.

Some women live with stable disease for many months, or even years, before the last available treatment loses effectiveness or becomes toxic to organs or other body systems and has to be discontinued.

At some point in this process, most women have to confront the fact that recurrent advanced ovarian cancer is likely to kill them.

Some, determined to live as long as possible, suffer through treatment after treatment, surgery after surgery, hospitalization after hospitalization, until they die from a bowel obstruction or some other system failure. I had one friend who took this path because she wanted as much time as possible with the people she loved, especially her young grandchildren. Her suffering seemed intolerable to me, but I understood and respected her choice.

Others, when they run out of tolerable options, terminate treatment and go into hospice care, in order to remain as comfortable as possible and savor their last days, weeks, or months. Another friend of mine chose this path. I saw her the day before she died. She was receiving oxygen and morphine for comfort. During my visit, a hospice volunteer was giving her a massage. Her last days were filled with constant loving attention from her family and closest friends. I felt that she died with dignity and grace.

In Oregon and Washington, there's a third alternative. A woman who is expected to die within six months can obtain a legal prescription so that she can end her life at a time of her own choosing. A third friend of mine danced her heart out one night at a concert, and she died the next day. I never knew if this was a coincidence or if she took advantage of the Oregon law, but either way it seemed like a great way to go, living with joy until the end.

I had two years of NED before my first recurrence. At that point I had to accept that I was not going to be one of the lucky few. After treatment, I got one more year of NED, and then started treatment for my second recurrence.

I've now been in treatment for eighteen consecutive months. During this time I've had several different kinds of chemotherapy. Some were ineffective for my particular cancer; others were effective but caused reactions or turned out to be toxic in other ways. My doctor has now said that he considers my cancer to be stable; he does not expect that I will again dance with NED. My current treatment is tolerable, and my cancer symptoms are manageable. As long as this remains the case, I will try to sustain this holding pattern.

But I've said from the beginning that quality of life was more important to me than having extra months, or even a year or two, of life without comfort or pleasure. For me, comfort means absence of pain or sickness. Pleasure means eating foods I enjoy, traveling, and doing photography. My favorite foods are ice cream, red meat, and junk food. I've been spending my retirement savings on small ship adventures (Baja California, Galápagos, Central America, and Arctic Svalbard) and photography workshops (Big Sur, Maine, Molokai, and Mexico). I spend my time at home planning and anticipating these trips, as well as editing, printing, and framing my photographs.

I still believe that I would rather die than live with pain, suffering, or the inability to enjoy my activities. At that point, I expect to terminate treatment and take advantage of the Oregon Death with Dignity law to end my life.

These have become the words I live by:

I will fight for my life as long as I have a life that feels worth fighting for. Then I will stop.

A Personal Perspective on Making Decisions about the End of Life

Marcy Westerling

I found out about my ovarian cancer through a collapsed lung, statistically an extremely negative predictor of survival. I understood I was terminally ill. Despite that clarity, I didn't address end-of-life planning. I was in front-line treatment, on a clinical trial; my focus was on staying alive.

Fear of death, panic attacks, and crying jags were companions those first months, and every decision I made, in retrospect, was really about impending death. I avoided paperwork as always, so instead made decisions about quality of life. Where did I want to live my closing years? What choices would best position me to live the most fully?

I moved from the country to the city. I had planned to stay in my country home for my final four decades, now I needed to think in terms of a final few years. The city offered the ease and services that facing death required.

I had to stop working even though I loved my job. I opted for an active volunteer role that gave me the best of stimulation and relevance without the burdens of employment I could no longer shoulder. I cherished my access to Social Security Disability Insurance and then Medicare, even as both choices required downsizing my life—you downsize as you face death. Right?

I created a simple yet full life. It was a post-cancer life. It is a pre-death life, but it is a life all about being fully alive for whatever time I have left.

Initially reading memoirs that described how others coped with such imminent mortality assisted me. My grief and panic lessened as I joined a club that I entitled "livingly dying" (co-opted from the late Christopher Hitchens)—being dedicated to life while holding your pink slip from the world. I founded a support group called It's a Dying Shame to allow terminally ill women the comfort of gathering in living rooms to process our emotions about this walk toward death. We laugh a lot. The group grows smaller.

As my first anniversary of diagnosis approached, I wrote to my inner circle of friends and detailed how I wanted my body handled. I had a vision, it mattered to me, and I felt relief once that was done.

I still have paperwork, but I have enough death decisions clarified to feel at peace. I live in a state that allows Death with Dignity, and I am informed on what I would need to line up should I choose that approach. I no longer feel fear about death; instead I allow myself to accept the sadness at saying goodbye early. I reserve my final stage of grief for my final stage of life—the active dying stage of no more treatment options. I am not there today.

CHAPTER 15

Decisions at the End of Life

F. J. Montz, MD, KM, FACOG, FACS

A n anecdote from Rick provides one perspective on the value of self-determination as a person approaches the end of life: "Recently, my sixteen-year-old son, Rocky, and I saw a movie that was the most popular movie in America the week it was released. The movie lacked plot and character development, but it was great adolescent-boy entertainment and almost worth the seventeen dollars I had to pay for us to get in. There was one line in the flick that was worth remembering and, believe it or not, is quite appropriate to mention in this chapter. Two action-hero brothers are off to engage in righteous battle. Before they charge into the horde of bad guys, they look each other in the eye and scowl, 'Live free, die well.' Pretty trite, huh? And, I think most of us would also say, not a bad motto to live and die by."

We are not going to address the issue of living free, though that wouldn't be a bad topic for an entire book about how to deal with cancer. But we do need to spend some time talking about dying well. The discussion is divided into two sections, one on end-of-life decisions (this chapter) and the other on death (the next chapter). From a time-line perspective, we will talk about what happens from the time a disease becomes incurable to the time the heart and lungs stop—when a medical professional would be willing to verify death. Just as we are going to avoid the issue of what it means to live free, we are going to avoid a big discussion about when someone actually dies, though we probably all have our own opinions about when that is.

In this chapter we focus on how patients make decisions about what happens up until the terminal event and thereafter. For a discussion of the issues that can be controlled in and around the moment of death, see chapter 16.

Here's another story from Rick's experience that illustrates the importance of an open dialogue between the patient and her caregivers when treatment options have run out:

Not long ago I had to do one of the most painful and at the same time one of the most personally rewarding things that I do as a cancer doc. I had to keep a promise to Dana F. and share with her, one of my long-time patients, the reality that despite all I had tried to do for her, we really had run out of options. Curing her disease had long ago fallen away as a potential option. And now, even our ability to meaningfully prolong her life had evaporated.

When I had first met Dana three years before, she had been a healthy and active professional woman who was director of sales for a large national organization. She was married to a great guy, Ben, and they had a charming son the same age as one of my sons. To bond us even more tightly, she and her husband were both big-time motorcycle enthusiasts, and I shared this hobby.

Friday morning Dana and I decided to make one last-ditch effort to surgically develop a way to repeatedly evacuate the mucous material that her disease was producing. We hoped she could then get some relief from her pressure-related symptoms of abdominal distension and the unrelenting nausea that wasn't being controlled with any antiemetic protocol we could come up with. Unfortunately, I wasn't able to accomplish much in the operating room, and now we had to deal with the issue of what Dana would want to do.

I had made a promise to Dana, as I do to all my patients, that if the time came when her disease was not curable and there was really nothing more that we could do that had a legitimate chance of helping prolong her life in a meaningful way, I would tell her (and any family members she wanted me to), so that her personal preferences would be preeminent in her decision-making process. When I left the operating room, I met with Dana's husband. During our forty-five minutes together, I shared with Ben the findings of the surgery and the reality that we had run out of treatment options. He and I discussed the need to make sure that everyone who needed to be involved was fully informed about what was going on and was supportive of letting Dana make her own self-directed but data-based decisions.

The time Ben and I spent together while Dana was settling into the recovery room was accompanied by two sets of wet eyes. This number grew to three sets when I had a similar discussion with Dana and Ben in Dana's room later that evening. We talked about what was going on, and Dana asked informed and specific questions, which I answered to the best of my ability. There was much else that we shared, and the process of making end-of-life decisions went from a general "This is what I want" to a very specific "These are the issues I am facing today and tomorrow (and I hope the day beyond this), and this is exactly what I want done and why."

The biggest end-of-life decisions are the decisions regarding what an individual wants to do with the time she or he has left and where and with whom the person wants to spend that time. Before people can make decisions about what they want to do with the end of their lives, however, they need to be fully aware and understand that they are coming to the end of their lives. This statement may sound ridiculous, but recent scientific investigations have shown that we health care professionals are not as forthright and open with our patients (all of whom have placed their trust in us that we will be honest) as we should be in sharing with them the truth about their disease and life expectancy.

Though some of this "failure to disclose" is a response to an expressed or implied "failure to want to know" (that is, the patient tells the health care provider or otherwise lets the provider know that he or she does not want to know the truth), much of it is a result of the emotional pain that health care professionals feel when they have to confess, first to themselves, and then to the patient, that neither of them is going to get the preferred outcome (semipermanent reestablishment of patient wellness).

We find it extremely hard to tell someone that she is going to die and that we (and the body of scientific knowledge and the health system that we represent) have failed her. We share our inner emotions and feelings of inadequacy at not being able to facilitate the "saving of a life" with only a very small percentage of our patients, but we tell almost all our patients how much it means to us that they trust us with their lives. As Rick has said in the past (and as was captured on camera and then broadcast on the television documentary *Hopkins 24/7*), it never ceases to amaze him how young women who are dying will try to make *him* feel better when he confesses to them that he believes he has failed them.

What Do You Want to Do with the Time You Have Left?

Rick said, "I ask my patients this question point blank. I need to relieve my own conscience that I have brought the issue up and that they have heard this from me." *What do you want to do with the time you have left?*

Do you want to spend your time being treated with therapies that have a very low rate of response but a well-known, predictable, and documented rate of toxicity? Do you want to take a trip, go visit someone, accomplish something special? Is there a unique event that you want so much to attend that you are willing to try almost anything to make it to the event? A wedding, a Bar Mitzvah, the birth of a grandchild, or something similar?

Part of the answer to this question involves a person's attitude toward "going gently into that good night." The range of attitudes in this regard is truly remarkable. The following is an example from Rob's practice:

Rob recently had a patient whose disease recurred quickly. The patient was reoperated on and repeatedly retreated. No matter what was done, the disease just kept growing, and the future and the time line had become certain. Despite significant persistent side effects of her treatments, which were added to the effects of progressive disease, she just wanted to keep going at it. We were running out of drugs to use, a situation that is very uncommon. This patient eventually died from a combination of progressive disease and toxicity of treatment. But to the end she was asking for more. And what was uniquely amazing about this exemplary woman was not that she wanted to keep going at life—something we often see in young women who have many life challenges and tasks ahead of them—but that she was approaching the average age of death for American women. Although she was interested in seeing a new grandchild born, that wasn't the real motivator. What motivated her was simply a personal code that she was "never going to give up."

Of course, this is an unusual case. More commonly, women decide that they have reached a point where they have had enough and just want to be left alone. They want quality, not quantity, and are willing to do a lot to get that quality.

One of our "rules to practice by" is never to assume how a patient will answer a question. This credo should be applied to *every* decision, whether active or by default, that a patient can make, but it is never more crucial in the natural history of a woman with ovarian cancer than when she is making end-of-life decisions. Every change in medication, every new blood test ordered, every visit that is scheduled, must be done in association with the patient's verbal confirmation: "This is what I want done." When there is little time left, it is incredibly important that every minute be spent in a way that is completely consistent with the patient's wishes.

Where and with Whom Do You Want to Spend the Time You Have Left?

Several specific questions need to be considered by patients who are facing the end of life.

Where Do You Want to Die?

With the wide availability of home hospice in the United States, there is no reason a patient can't receive all her health care and services to relieve suffering at home—services that until the 1980s were generally available only in the inpatient setting. So from the perspective of quality of life, there should be no difference between spending one's last days at home or in a hospital. In all honesty, however, this lack of difference exists only in an ideal world. In the real world, where there are insurance and resource limitations, it may be difficult for a given individual to receive the same care at home as in a hospital. This should not be the case, but unfortunately, it often is.

There are, of course, many people who don't want to die at home. Certain religious traditions have taboos about the spirits of dead individuals and where they are released when the body dies. Some patients do not want family members to bear the memory of a dead body in the house. And there are other reasons that a person may not want to die in her home or in the home of a friend or family member. Whether *we* find the reasons rational doesn't matter: to the patient, these reasons are real and valid. We need to respect the reasons fully and help the patient spend her last days where she chooses, if at all possible.

How Alert Do You Want to Be?

Though one of the goals of optimal pain relief is to relieve pain to the greatest degree possible while maintaining functionality, there are some times, as death approaches, when there is a trade-off between total pain control and total alertness. Some patients are willing to deal with low or even moderate degrees of pain if doing so means they can have maximum alertness. For some individuals, even the slightest amount of pain is too much; they might say that if elimi-

nating all pain means some sleepiness and lack of ability to be atten-
tive, so be it. Health care providers need to address these issues and
have an open and frank discussion leading to an understanding with
the patient.

Do You Want to Be Intubated or Have Cardiopulmonary Resuscitation?

This question would only come into consideration if the patient
"coded" (short for Code Blue, the traditional voice page that used to
be called when a patient stopped breathing or lost a pulse or blood
pressure). The implied obligation of a health care professional in this
situation, unless explicitly informed otherwise, is to keep a patient
"alive" until even the most heroic efforts have failed.

It was demonstrated in the 1980s that when people with a terminal disease "code," few of them leave the intensive care unit alive.
Also, a person who is in the intensive care unit (where she must be
if she is intubated and on a ventilator or is receiving certain medications) is physically isolated from those people who matter to her
most. Even if a patient has chosen to die at home, she is not protected
from being taken to the hospital and intubated and aggressively re-
suscitated, unless she provides specific instructions to the contrary.
An example:

> One Sunday evening when Rick was covering the Kelly
> Gynecologic Oncology Service, he received a call from the
> daughter of one of his partner's patients, Marion S., who had
> decided to die at home. The daughter described to Rick the
> pattern of her mother's breathing and said that her mom
> was not very responsive. The daughter wanted to know what
> she should do. Even though Marion had explicitly stated her
> desire to die at home and not to undergo heroic attempts
> at resuscitation, and had made this clear to her daughter
> and family, if the daughter had called 911, the paramedics
> would have performed CPR and transferred Marion to the
> nearest hospital unless there was a written and valid "Do not
> resuscitate" order.
>
> Understandably, Marion's daughter was scared. Rick spent a

few minutes going over the issues with her and summarizing both her mother's wishes and what might happen over the next few hours. Fortunately, Marion fell deeper into sleep and literally passed to the beyond in her home, with the person she loved the most in the whole world (and who in return loved Marion the most) at her side.

There are many ways of making sure that a person's wishes regarding heroic measures are respected. Probably the best way is to execute a *living will*, which is a legal instrument that explicitly states what an individual wants done (and does not want done) at the end of life. We strongly encourage every one of our patients to complete one of these documents and have it notarized, and then to give copies of the document to family members, friends, health care professionals, lawyers, and so on. The more people who have copies of the living will, the better the situation.

Another legal instrument, similar but distinct, is the *durable power of attorney for health care*. In this legal document, people designate the individual or individuals who will serve as a surrogate for them, making health care decisions for them if they are unable to do so. The durable power of attorney for health care does not specify what is going to be done; it only designates who is going to make the decisions about what will be done if the patient cannot. Rick explained, "Both Kate and I have living wills and durable powers of attorney for health care. We have designated each other as surrogates, and we have named alternates (friends, brothers, and so forth) as well. Interestingly, our living wills are different as to what we want done . . . but that is another story altogether!"

What Do You Want Done with Your Mortal Remains? What Kind of Funeral or Wake or Party or Ceremony Do You Want Taking Place after You Die?

This decision can be made at any time during one's life and therefore is not necessarily an end-of-life decision, but it becomes increasingly timely as one comes closer to death. Here's a personal example that Rick offered:

One of the most interesting discussions I ever had with my parents occurred in the business-class cabin of a US Airways airplane between Philadelphia and Munich one fall. I like to take trips with my parents every year or two, serving as part tour guide, part caregiver. One fall they wanted to go back to Italy, where they had lived for a couple of years in their early twenties shortly after World War II. We flew together, my parents sitting beside each other and me in the seat behind. After we were "at our cruising altitude," and the pilot had turned off the "fasten seat belt" sign, I moved up and sat on the floor in front of my parents. We were just chitchatting, and the fact came up that these 78-year-olds had both visited the mortician to make decisions regarding what they wanted done if they should die. With a little prodding, they shared their decisions.

My mom wanted to be cremated, have her ashes put in a nice urn (the cheapest one the mortician showed them was five hundred bucks!), and have a nice memorial service (funeral) in her local church followed by a "lunch." My dad also wanted to be cremated, though he didn't want to spend the money on the urn (we decided that a Folgers pound-and-a-half coffee can would work nicely . . . Thanks, Coen brothers), wasn't into the church and reception thing, and agreed that the family could go out to dinner together afterward but that I had to pay for it, and the cost couldn't be charged against his estate. He wanted his ashes spread across the prairies and upper Missouri River, an area where he had lived for more than forty-seven years. Because my parents thought about what they wanted and shared their wishes with me (my mom actually wrote hers down and noted what songs she wanted to have sung and what readings she was interested in), I can do my best to make sure that their wishes are respected.

Just as with the living will and the durable power of attorney for health care, it is a good idea to decide whether you have any strongly held wishes about funerals, body management, flowers, and other details. Write your wishes down and tell the people you trust about them.

CHAPTER 16

Death and the Process of Dealing with Loss

F. J. Montz, MD, KM, FACOG, FACS

~~~~~~

W hen is a person dead? Although the legal system has given us code after code as a result of difficult tort cases, the definition of death still seems elusive. A couple of stories from Rick inform our reflections:

My mom's dad had multiple medical problems before he died. He had a primary gastric cancer (I still remember being in the patient waiting area at St. Luke's Hospital in Cedar Rapids, Iowa, when we visited him as he recovered from his subtotal gastrectomy). However, being of tough immigrant Nordic-Deutsch stock, his body wouldn't give up yet. Unfortunately, he was severely impaired both mentally and physically as a result of multiple strokes. The last eighteen or so months of his life were spent receiving full-time "nursing" care in his home, supplied by his wife of almost sixty years, my grandmother, Emma Meier Stolte. During that time there really didn't appear to be much left of that incredibly strong Germanic farmer other than a frail and marginally functional body.

Grandpa Stolte died when I was 16 and unquestionably still

developing my own personal worldview (still am, my wife, Kate, would say). When my grandfather died, my grandmother didn't outwardly show much sign of loss. I remember her commenting on that very fact in my presence. What she said has stuck with me: "Emil died when he was no longer able to communicate with me. I did most of my grieving then."

A few days ago I was walking outside between buildings at the Johns Hopkins Hospital and Medical Institutions campus (as I like to do, to avoid staying inside the hospital buildings and blasting down hallways full of processed air), returning to my academic office from the Weinberg Building, having completed my second of three major surgeries for the day. I was tumbling over in my mind all the issues I was dealing with at that time, but mostly weighing family closeness against career. Out of nowhere, my grandfather Montz (known as Doc) was with me. Something had made me remember him and think about his unyielding commitment to just and high-quality patient care. I felt that if I had wanted to, I could have picked up a phone and called him to ask his sage (and quite opinionated and probably profane) advice. Although Doc had been physically dead for twenty-three years, longer than I have been a doctor, he was very, very alive.

These two stories (without even mentioning the Christian concept of eternal life) touch on the question "When are we dead?" In more spiritual and humanistic realms, the answer might be "It depends."

By legal and medical statute and convention, death occurs at the moment when there is no longer measurable cardiac activity. In a setting away from health facilities or cardiac monitoring, this is said to be the time when there is no longer a detectable pulse or heart pumping. If monitoring is occurring, a person is considered to be dead when there is no longer measurable cardiac electric activity on a monitor (electrocardiogram).

There is some value in understanding the concept of *brain death,* the situation in which the person has cardiopulmonary function (as a result of either natural function or artificial support) but a series of accepted tests have demonstrated that the brain is not working at all, even on a reflexive basis. Tests to determine brain death are usually done so that artificial support of cardiac or pulmonary function can be removed. Of course, patients need to be in the hospital to receive this support (usually in an intensive care unit, or ICU), and it is there that a decision is made whether to continue what would be considered futile efforts.

In fifteen years as an attending gynecologic oncologist, Rick remembered only two instances when it was necessary to make a determination about brain death so as to withdraw cardiopulmonary support. Neither of the women had a malignancy, but both had suffered codes and had been through a long period during which their brains didn't get much or any oxygen. A strict protocol for determining brain death (which had been developed by the medical faculty and approved by both the legal office and the ethics committee of the institutions where he was practicing) was followed before pulmonary support was withdrawn. Withdrawing pulmonary support means stopping the respirator that is keeping the lungs working and is causing oxygen to go into the blood of the patient; this action is sometimes called "pulling the plug," a term that comes from the idea of stopping the electricity that runs through the mechanical ventilator. After the respirator was stopped, the tube in the patient's throat was gently removed. Cardiac monitoring continued until all electrical activity stopped, something that took only a few moments in both cases. These patients, whom Rick had cared for and cared about, were now dead.

Why does death frighten us so much? For most modern people who do not hold any of the traditional medieval beliefs about a physical purgatory or hell, psychologists tell us that the fear of death is not fear of what is on "the other side" but concerns about losing something valuable and about what will happen to those we care about once we are gone. Many of our patients, having accomplished all that they had hoped for in their lives, and seeing the people and things that mattered most to them either precede them in death or lose meaning, have looked forward to death, even longed for it. They had nothing to lose, nothing to worry about, and were anxious to "get on." Most often these are older people, and many have just recently lost a long-time life mate. We all know examples of these couples. Recently an individual who was a major influence in Rick's life was in this situation:

> Burt N. was my high school civics teacher. He was a great guy, trying to make the most out of what was mostly a group of marginally talented and motivated kids. Burt always did it in a respectful way and often taught some simple though incredibly valuable lessons along the way. I will never forget a sign he hung in his office. It said: "If you think that you are irreplaceable, just put your fist into a bucket of water and then pull it out. You are as difficult to replace as it was to fill the hole left in the water when you removed your hand." That one has stayed with me.
>
> Burt and his wife had been married more than fifty years, had raised five kids, and had seen them all move out of the state. As they got into their late seventies, they sold their house and moved into an assisted living complex close to my parents. Though both were in good health for folks of their age, Burt got a bad cold and quickly died. Six weeks later his life mate, who had nothing physically wrong with her, was gone too. She had lived her life and had had enough. In some metaphysical way I know that these two individuals, who at least outwardly appeared to be so tightly bound to each other, are together.

Most of the women who are our patients are not at a place in their lives where they are willing to stop living. Many have resolved issues of loss and separation, but few desire death. Rick and his wife had a relevant experience:

> Kate once underwent an evaluation and was noted to have an X-ray finding that was suspicious for the presence of an aggressive form of uterine cancer. A diagnostic procedure needed to be performed to determine whether a malignancy was present. As the day of the procedure came closer and closer, Kate became less anxious as I became more. What had happened? Well, Kate had made me promise that, if something happened to her, I would give up my seventy-hour-a-week work style plus frequent travel and focus on the care of our kids.

Once I had unhesitatingly agreed to do just that, Kate, knowing that my conscience would make me keep my word, had less concern about what would happen to those she would leave and was more comfortable with the future. I, on the other hand, realized that I could potentially be losing two of the three most valued "things" in my life: my soul-mate life partner and my mission-driven career. I feared the unknown and the loss of something that was immeasurably valuable. Happily, no cancer was present. Kate was successfully treated, and normality was reestablished.

This vignette illustrates a point: it is the loss of that which we value that makes death frightening.

Death is something that cancer doctors must become accustomed to but should never become comfortable with. If the death of one of our patients fails to sadden us, we have lost that critical gift of caring that made us worthy of being labeled doctors (and the same goes for nurses). Caring for dying people must always be painful; it can never become routine. Every time one of our patients dies, no matter how close or distant our emotional attachment is to him or her, a small part of us dies as well. It is one of those great mysteries of the human spirit that we can repeatedly die yet still have more to give. This miracle falls into that category which includes a parent's endless love and a soldier's endless courage.

As we discussed in chapter 15, we encourage our patients, even when they are fighting their hardest to live, to reflect on their death. Where do they want to be? Whom do they want to be with? What do they want to have happen afterward regarding donation of body parts, cremation or burial, memorial services, and celebrations of life? Whom do they want inheriting whatever temporal possessions or resources they have? Whom do they want taking over for them (not replacing them!) in their roles in the family and community? Even thinking about these issues can be paralyzingly painful for some women. However, these issues really must be addressed.

Elisabeth Kübler-Ross, in her landmark book *On Death and Dying*, describes how dealing with loss is a process. The process of dealing with loss is as important as reaching the end goal of acceptance.

Most people require professional help in dealing with the concepts of loss and death. We strongly encourage our patients, early in their disease process, to develop a relationship with an individual or individuals who can help them through the process of coping with the idea of their own death. This person may be a pastor, priest, or rabbi; a psychologist; a social worker; or a counselor. Support group therapy (such as the therapy available at Wellness Communities) can often be helpful. Taking an active approach, at the woman's own pace and with support from others, makes it likely that she will be prepared if she faces death. We hope that death will not be the eventual outcome of ovarian cancer. However, should it be, the woman will be best prepared if the issues surrounding the end of life and death have been addressed and processed.

CHAPTER 17

Survivorship

F. J. Montz, MD, KM, FACOG, FACS

〜〜〜〜〜〜〜〜〜〜〜〜〜〜〜〜〜〜〜〜〜〜〜〜〜〜〜〜〜〜〜〜〜

If it is relatively easy, within the limitations we have discussed, to define when one dies, shouldn't it be easy to define when one is surviving? Well, guess what? It isn't. If you define surviving using purely biological criteria, well, then, yes, surviving is not being dead. But surviving is so much more than that! Ideally, it is being intellectually, spiritually, and physically fully functional. And we love to aim for the ideal.

As we pointed out earlier in this book, the stress of the diagnosis and treatment of ovarian cancer can push marginally functional relationships over the edge. The same holds true for everything we are and do. A person may be willing to put up with a barely acceptable job, for example, until she looks death in the eye, realizes that life is a limited commodity, and says, "Take this job and shove it"—to quote the old country and western song. What about interpersonal relationships? How she spends her leisure time? What she does with money? And on and on . . .

Dealing with ovarian cancer can remarkably change what a person is satisfied with and how she wants to live her life. It actually allows—or forces—people to address issues they have never addressed before. We have seen many women come out on the other side of their initial cancer treatment happier and more fulfilled than when they entered, because they had decided that taking stock of their lives and actively managing them was essential. (See the story of Inez V., below.) Unfortunately, women can also come out on the other side of their initial ovarian cancer treatment a total emotional, intellectual, and physical wreck, paralyzed by fear about when the cancer would come back and angry at everyone about everything. Here are two stories. One is a story of how not to survive; the other is a story of how to survive.

> Isabel P. was diagnosed with ovarian cancer in her early seventies and underwent all the appropriate therapies. Fortunately, she fell into that group of ladies whose disease goes into remission. But she was suffering more after her treatment than she ever had before. She was angry at God for having done this to her. She had decided to leave her long-term home and move closer to where her children lived . . . and she *hated* her new home. She said she didn't have any friends, didn't like the weather, and so on. And even though she had regained her strength, she couldn't sleep at night because she was so afraid the cancer would come back. She said there were days when she just wished she were dead (a professional mental health worker called in by Isabel's doctor determined that Isabel did not pose a risk to herself). Isabel P. was *not surviving,* although she was very much alive and would be for a significant time to come, barring an accident or sudden death from some other medical problem.

> Inez V., too, was diagnosed with ovarian cancer and had all the standard therapies. Her story is similar to Isabel P.'s, except for one factor: Inez's disease recurred about five months after she completed initial therapy. Not long after that, her life partner of eighteen years died of a heart attack. Yet Inez decided that she was going to listen to the wake-up call she had received from the ovarian cancer. She was going to control her life and try to be as happy as possible for as long as possible. She joined a yoga program at the local Wellness Community, started watercolor

painting (something she had been doing on and off her whole life but had let slip to the sidelines while she was raising her children and working), and was enjoying lunching with friends (though in a modest way, since, she confessed, her retirement benefits were limited). She joyfully painted a wonderful still life that hangs in the director's conference room of our department. Inez V. realized that her life was short, and though she was sad when she thought that she would likely die before her grandkids graduated from college or married—events she had hoped to attend—she was grateful for every day she had and for the limited nature of the suffering she had experienced to date.

Which of these two ladies is surviving? We would suggest that Inez V., who is actively dying, is the one who is surviving, while Isabel P., who has no physical, chemical, or radioactive evidence of disease, is not surviving.

Really, it has to do with how you define *survivorship*. We discussed some of these issues in chapter 16, but there is value in reviewing them. Life is a terminal disease process, and we all will eventually physically die. And though there are lots of folks who believe and who will tell you that there is an "eternal life," few Americans believe that this eternal life is going to be much like what our everyday lives are like. Therefore, most of us believe that when you die, you (that physical you that can be described in height, weight, and hair and eye color, but also the personality you) are not going to exist in any way that resembles the you whom your family and friends know. For the people we know as ourselves, this time may well be the only time around.

But what about life, and survivorship? Just having a heartbeat and breathing, or even having cognitive thought, may on a certain level constitute life, but they don't define *survival*. Survival is finding joy in the world around us, even when our lives are not necessarily the way we want them to be. Being productive and useful, even when we may not be able to do all that we used to be able to do or all that we could have done. Having a meaning and serving a purpose for others. That is survivorship!

Since September 2001, many pundits have talked about how much of the financial and moral degeneration that has occurred is really our own fault. We Americans, they claim, have become very "me focused." What is in it *for me?* How can I get ahead—get more money, possessions, fame, power? Sadly, generation after generation and life story after life story have demonstrated that when we focus on what is measurable (bank account balances, number of cars, cost of the latest piece of clothing) rather than on what is immeasurable (who cares for us and whom do we care for? how much are we putting back into the community?), we are condemned to be unhappy, because we are never going to be able to get enough. Remember that old appellation "poor little rich girl"?

Being alive is having meaning and making a difference. Let's answer this question: If an individual is totally isolated from the rest of the world, never, ever interacting in any way and having absolutely no impact on anyone else's life, so that no one knows that she or he exists, *does* she or he exist?

No one can argue that the personality we were born with makes no difference in how we view our situation, how good or bad we consider our lives to be. Different patients will respond differently to the diagnosis and treatment of ovarian cancer because they have different personalities. What we are talking about in this chapter, however, is our desire to help our patients toward survivorship, even taking personality differences into account.

When a patient of ours is having difficulty finding any pleasure in life (a condition called *anhedonia*), we, as health care professionals, must first take steps to find out whether she is clinically depressed. One who is depressed might respond very well to having focused care from an experienced mental health provider. If the patient is not depressed but is still having a difficult time of it, we try to counsel her, talking about some of the ideas in this chapter.

It is most important to recognize where the "comfort zone" of survivorship is for you as an individual. Not everyone can be as proactive and engaged in life as Inez V.; however, no one should suffer as much and be as disconnected from life as Isabel P. Ovarian cancer is a traumatizing illness, no question about it. It is an illness that requires treatment not only of the cancer, but of the whole person as well. True survivorship is something that can be defined only by you, as you consider your unique personal feelings and life goals. Recognizing that you are out of your comfort zone, and allowing your doctor and other health care professionals, family and friends, or clergy to help, can be the first steps toward really "surviving" ovarian cancer.

Each woman diagnosed with ovarian cancer will have her own, very personal definition of survivorship, and the particulars of how she navigates that journey are equally unique to her as an individual. In general terms, however, a large component of "surviving" ovarian cancer has to do with being in control of one's life as much as possible, and with being as "well" (in all aspects of Wellness) as possible, and with finding joy and pleasure in living life to the fullest extent possible. This book is not intended to be an instruction book that will work for everyone. Instead, we provide it as a guide, a resource to help patients define their own path to surviving ovarian cancer and beyond.

Resources

American Cancer Society (ACS)
250 Williams Street NW
Atlanta, Georgia, 30303
1-800-ACS-2345
www.cancer.org

American Society of Clinical Oncology
(ASCO)
2318 Mill Road, Suite 800
Alexandria, VA 22314
571-483-1780 or 888-651-3038
www.cancer.net

CancerCare
275 Seventh Avenue
New York, NY 10001
212-302-2400
1-800-813-HOPE
www.cancercare.org

Cancer Support Community
1050 17th Street NW, Suite 500
Washington, DC 20036
202-659-9709 or 1-888-793-9355
www.cancersupportcommunity.org

Familial Ovarian Cancer Registry
Roswell Park Cancer Institute
Elm and Carlton Streets
Buffalo, NY 14263
1-800-OVARIAN
www.ovariancancer.com

The International Ovarian Cancer
Connection
P.O. Box 7948
Amarillo, TX 79114-7948
210-401-1604
conversations@ovarian-news.org
www.ovarian-news.com

Look Good Feel Better
Personal Care Products Council
Foundation
1620 L Street NW, 12th Floor
Washington, DC 20036
1-800-395-LOOK
www.lookgoodfeelbetter.org

National Cancer Institute (NCI)
1-800-4-Cancer
www.cancer.gov
www.cancer.gov/cancerinfo/coping

National Coalition for Cancer
Survivorship
1010 Wayne Avenue, Suite 315
Silver Spring, MD 20910-5600
877-622-7937
www.canceradvocacy.org

National Ovarian Cancer Coalition
(NOCC)
2501 Oak Lawn Avenue, Suite 435
Dallas, TX 75219
1-888-OVARIAN
www.ovarian.org

The Neuropathy Association
110 W. 40th Street, Suite 1804
New York, NY 10018
212-692-0662
www.neuropathy.org

Oncology Nursing Society
125 Enterprise Drive
Pittsburgh, PA 15275
866-257-4ONS
www.ons.org

Ovarian Cancer Canada
416-962-2700 or 1-877-413-7970
www.ovariancanada.org

Ovarian Cancer National Alliance
1101 14th Street NW, Suite 850
Washington, DC 20005
202-331-1332 or 866-399-6262
www.ovariancancer.org

Ovarian Cancer Research Fund (OCRF)
14 Pennsylvania Plaza, Suite 1710
New York, NY 10122
1-800-873-9569
www.ocrf.org

Patient Advocate Foundation (PAF)
421 Butler Farm Road
Hampton, VA 23666
1-800-532-5274
www.patientadvocate.org

SHARE: Self-Help for Women with
    Breast or Ovarian Cancer
1501 Broadway, Suite 704A
New York, NY 10036
212-719-0364
866-891-2392
www.sharecancersupport.org

Society of Gynecologic Oncology
230 W. Monroe Street, Suite 710
Chicago, IL 60606-4703
1-800-444-4441
www.sgo.org

Notes

Chapter 1. What Is Ovarian Cancer?

1. Kurman RJ, Shih I-M, The origin and pathogenesis of epithelial ovarian cancer: a proposed unifying theory, *Am J Surg Pathol* 2010; 34:433–443.

2. Guth U, Huang DJ, Bauer G, et al., Metastatic patterns at autopsy in patients with ovarian carcinoma, *Cancer* 2007; 110:1272–1280.

3. Howlader N, Noone AM, Krapcho M, et al. (eds), SEER Cancer Statistics Review, 1975–2011, National Cancer Institute, Bethesda, MD, http://seer.cancer .gov/csr/1975_2011/, based on November 2013 SEER data submission, posted to the SEER website April 2014.

4. Howlader N, Noone AM, Krapcho M, et al. (eds), SEER Cancer Statistics Review, 1975–2009 (Vintage 2009 Populations), National Cancer Institute, Bethesda, MD, http://seer.cancer.gov/csr/1975_2009_pops09/, based on November 2011 SEER data submission, posted to the SEER website April 2012, http:// seer.cancer.gov/csr/1975_2009_pops09/results_single/sect_01_table.01.pdf.

5. LCWK10, Deaths, Percent of Total Deaths, and Rank Order for 113 Selected Causes of Death, by Race and Sex: United States, 2001–2013, CDC/NCHS, National Vital Statistics System, Mortality 2013, www.cdc.gov/nchs/nvss/mor tality/lcwk10.htm.

6. Sharma A, Gentry-Maharaj A, Burnell M, et al., Assessing the malignant potential of ovarian inclusion cysts in postmenopausal women within the UK Collaborative Trial of Ovarian Cancer Screening (UKCTOCS): a prospective cohort study, *BJOG* 2011; 119:207–219.

7. Pothuri B, Leitao MM, Levine DA, et al., Genetic analysis of the early natural history of epithelial ovarian carcinoma, *PLoS One* 2010; 5:e10358.

8. Callahan MJ, Crum CP, Medeiros F, et al., Primary fallopian tube malignancies in BRCA-positive women undergoing surgery for ovarian cancer risk reduction, *J Clin Oncol* 2007; 25:3985–3990.

9. Carcangiu ML, Radice P, Manoukian S, et al., Atypical epithelial proliferation in fallopian tubes in prophylactic salpingo-oophorectomy specimens from BRCA1 and BRCA2 germline mutation carriers, *Int J Gynecol Pathol* 2004; 23:35–40.

10. Colgan TJ, Murphy J, Cole DE, et al., Occult carcinoma in prophylactic oophorectomy specimens: prevalence and association with BRCA germline mutation status, *Am J Surg Pathol* 2001; 25:1283–1289.

11. Finch A, Shaw P, Rosen B, et al., Clinical and pathologic findings of prophylactic salpingo-oophorectomies in 159 BRCA1 and BRCA2 carriers, *Gynecol Oncol* 2006; 100:58–64.

12. Medeiros F, Muto MG, Lee Y, et al., The tubal fimbria is a preferred site for early adenocarcinoma in women with familial ovarian cancer syndrome, *Am J Surg Pathol* 2006; 30:230–236.

13. Paley PJ, Swisher EM, Garcia RL, et al., Occult cancer of the fallopian tube in BRCA-1 germline mutation carriers at prophylactic oophorectomy: a case for recommending hysterectomy at surgical prophylaxis, *Gynecol Oncol* 2001; 80:176–180.

14. Shaw PA, Rouzbahman M, Pizer ES, et al., Candidate serous cancer precursors in fallopian tube epithelium of BRCA1/2 mutation carriers, *Mod Pathol* 2009; 22:1133–1138.

15. Piek JM, van Diest PJ, Zweemer RP, et al., Dysplastic changes in prophylactically removed fallopian tubes of women predisposed to developing ovarian cancer, *J Pathol* 2001; 195:451–456.

16. Kindelberger DW, Lee Y, Miron A, et al., Intraepithelial carcinoma of the fimbria and pelvic serous carcinoma: evidence for a causal relationship, *Am J Surg Pathol* 2007; 31:161–169.

17. Pearce CL, Templeman C, Rossing MA, et al., Association between endometriosis and risk of histological subtypes of ovarian cancer: a pooled analysis of case-control studies, *Lancet Oncol* 2012; 13:385–394.

18. Chen S, Parmigiani G, Meta-analysis of BRCA1 and BRCA2 penetrance, *J Clin Oncol* 2007; 25:1329–1333.

19. Rossouw JE, Anderson GL, Prentice RL, et al., Risks and benefits of estrogen plus progestin in healthy postmenopausal women: principal results from the Women's Health Initiative randomized controlled trial, *JAMA* 2002; 288:321–333.

20. Menon U, Gentry-Maharaj A, et al., Sensitivity and specificity of multimodal and ultrasound screening for ovarian cancer, and stage distribution of detected cancers: results of the prevalence screen of the UK Collaborative Trial of Ovarian Cancer Screening (UKCTOCS). *Lancet Oncol* 2009; 10:327–340.

21. Moyer VA, on behalf of the US Preventive Services Task Force, Risk assessment, genetic counseling, and genetic testing for BRCA-related cancer in women: U.S. Preventive Services Task Force recommendation statement, *Ann Intern Med* 2014; 160:271–281.

22. Brown DL, Andreotti RF, Lee SI, et al., ACR appropriateness criteria ovarian cancer screening, *Ultrasound Q* 2010; 26:219–223.

23. Goff BA, Mandel LS, Melancon CH, et al., Frequency of symptoms of ovarian cancer in women presenting to primary care clinics, *JAMA* 2004; 291:2705.

24. Goff BA, Mandel LS, Drescher CW, et al., Development of an ovarian cancer symptom index: possibilities for earlier detection, *Cancer* 2007; 109:221.

25. Goff BA, Lowe KA, Kane JC, et al., Symptom triggered screening for ovarian cancer: a pilot study of feasibility and acceptability, *Gynecol Oncol* 2012; 124:230.

Contributors

ROBERT E. BRISTOW, MD, MBA, FACOG, FACS, is director of Gynecologic Oncology Services, the Philip J. DiSaia Chair of Gynecologic Oncology, chief of the Division of Gynecologic Oncology, and a professor of obstetrics and gynecology, University of California, Irvine, Medical Center.

TERRI L. CORNELISON, MD, PHD, FACOG, is associate director for clinical research, Office of Research on Women's Health, Office of the Director, National Institutes of Health, and an assistant professor of gynecology and obstetrics, Johns Hopkins Medical Institutions.

F. J. MONTZ, MD, KM, FACOG, FACS, was a professor of gynecology and obstetrics, surgery, and oncology, Johns Hopkins Hospital and Medical Institutions.

PAULA J. ANASTASIA, RN, MN, AOCN, is a gynecology-oncology clinical nurse specialist at Cedars-Sinai Medical Center in Los Angeles.

ANA MILENA ANGARITA AFRICANO, MD, is an international gynecologic oncology research fellow, Department of Gynecology and Obstetrics, Johns Hopkins Medical Institutions.

DEBORAH K. ARMSTRONG, MD, is director of the Breast and Ovarian Surveillance Service, Johns Hopkins Medical Institutions.

RAMEZ N. ESKANDER, MD, is an assistant professor in gynecologic oncology, University of California, Irvine, Medical Center.

AMANDA NICKLES FADER, MD, is director of the Kelly Gynecologic Oncology Service and an associate professor of gynecology and obstetrics, Johns Hopkins Medical Institutions.

MARIO JAVIER PINEDA, MD, PHD, is an assistant professor of obstetrics and gynecology, Division of Gynecologic Oncology, Robert H. Lurie Comprehensive Cancer Center of Northwestern University.

LESLIE M. RANDALL, MD, is an assistant professor in gynecologic oncology, Department of Obstetrics and Gynecology, University of California, Irvine, Medical Center.

RITU SALANI, MD, MBA, is an associate professor in gynecologic oncology, Department of Obstetrics and Gynecology, Ohio State University Wexner Medical Center.

DILJEET K. SINGH, MD, DRPH, is a gynecologic oncologist at the Robert H. Lurie Comprehensive Cancer Center of Northwestern University and an assistant professor of obstetrics and gynecology, Northwestern University Feinberg School of Medicine.

EDWARD TANNER, MD, is associate director of the F. J. Montz Fellowship in Gynecologic Oncology and an assistant professor of gynecology and obstetrics, Johns Hopkins Medical Institutions.

SHARON D. THOMPSON, BSN, OCN, is a nurse coordinator in the Department of Gynecology and Obstetrics, Kelly Gynecologic Oncology Service, Johns Hopkins Hospital.

KALA VISVANATHAN, MD, MBBS, FRACP, MHS, is director of the Clinical Cancer Genetics and Prevention Service at the Sidney Kimmel Comprehensive Cancer Center, Johns Hopkins School of Medicine, and an associate professor in the Department of Epidemiology and Medical Oncology, Johns Hopkins Bloomberg School of Public Health and Johns Hopkins School of Medicine.

ELIZABETH A. WILEY, MS, CGC, is a genetic counselor in the Clinical Cancer Genetics and Prevention Service, Johns Hopkins Medical Institutions.

RICHARD ZELLARS, MD, is a professor and chair in the Department of Radiation Oncology, Indiana University Hospital.

Index

anxiety/fear (*cont.*)
and, 174; integrative approaches to, 175, 176, 179; medications for, 83, 84, 144; sleep and, 148; among survivors, 193, 214, 215, 218, 220, 224, 225, 229, 230, 273
Anzemet (dolasetron), 83, 84
apoptosis, 5–6, 49, 62
appearance, 93, 184–85
appetite, 79, 114, 115, 117, 146, 169
aprepitant (oral Emend), 84
argon beam coagulator (ABC), 37
Arimidex (anastrozole), 60, 61
Aromasin (exemestane), 61
aromatase inhibitors, 61, 182
aromatherapy, 176, 177
ascites, 24, 33, 238, 249, 250–51
ashwagandha, 179
aspirin, 78, 81, 129
assisted-reproductive technology, 31
astragalus, 179
Ativan (lorazepam), 54, 83, 84, 85, 129
attitude, positive, 115, 152, 191
autonomy of patient, 28
Avastin (bevacizumab), 63, 244–45, 247
Ayurvedic medicine, 157, 159

Bacopa, 179
Bag Balm, 101
bathing/showering, 43, 77, 95, 96, 98
Benadryl (diphenhydramine), 54, 83
benzodiazepines, 83, 149. *See also* lorazepam
beta-carotene, 164–65, 166–67, 168
bevacizumab (Avastin), 63, 244–45, 247
biomarkers, 50, 175; for diagnosis, 15, 24–25 (*see also* CA-125 serum level); to predict chemotherapy effectiveness, 235; surveillance of, 216, 217–18; for treatment monitoring, 49, 56
biopsy, 81; breast, 26; ovarian, 31, 32, 61, 234
Biosil (orthosilicic acid), 185
Biotene, 72
bisacodyl (Correctol, Dulcolax), 88, 89
bisphosphonates, 187
black cohosh, 178
bleeding: anemia due to, 79; herbs and, 161; during intercourse, 141; medication-induced, 81, 129; patient education for, 81–82; rectal, 81, 90; during surgery, 41, 239–40; thrombocytopenia and, 80–81, 244; vaginal, 217
blood clotting: herb effects on, 161; hor-

monal therapy and, 61; postoperative, 43
blood pressure, 27, 122, 173, 263; high, 39, 131, 144, 245; low, 83, 103, 127, 129
blood tests, 15, 24, 25, 96, 183, 261; for anemia, 78–79; central access catheter for, 50; before/during chemotherapy, 50, 56, 75, 76; to monitor for disease recurrence, 214, 217–18, 232, 234; before surgery, 27; for treatment monitoring, 39, 49, 56, 57, 75; of vitamin D level, 120. *See also* CA-125 serum level
blood transfusions, 41, 53, 79–80, 239–40; allergic reaction to, 239–40; central access catheter for, 50–51; infection risk from, 79, 239
body mass index, 186
bone health, 61, 140–41, 187; osteoporosis, 120, 140, 141, 144, 187
bowel: injury to, 240–41, 245; obstruction of, 41–42, 87, 108, 116, 249–50, 253; prep of, for surgery, 28–29; rest for, 41, 250; wall of, cancer spread to, 29
bowel function, 18, 19, 36, 88, 90; postoperative, 41, 43. *See also* constipation; diarrhea
brain death, 267–68
brain-stimulating games, 100, 150
BRAT diet, 45, 92, 125
BRCA gene mutations, 9, 11, 12, 198–99, 207–9, 210, 233; olaparib for carriers of, 245–46
Breast and Ovarian Surveillance Service (BOSS), 17
breast cancer, 7; BRCA gene mutations and, 11, 12, 198–99, 207–9; hormonal therapy for, 60; HRT and, 13, 140, 144; lifestyle and outcomes of, 157–58; male, 209; mind-body interventions for, 175; overweight and, 227; progesterone and, 12; screening for, 7, 14, 19, 26, 228; self-image and, 181–82; sleep and, 176; soy and, 165–66; TDM-1 for, 63–64; vaginal atrophy and, 141
breastfeeding, 8, 9, 12
breathing techniques, 21, 87, 152, 175, 176
bruising, 80–82
bupropion, 227

caffeine intake, 55, 92, 176, 222
calcium, 115, 120, 141; supplements of, 87, 98, 120, 187
calcium channel blockers, 161

caloric intake, 29, 36, 111, 114, 115–18, 121, 163, 186, 250

Camtosar (irinotecan), 91, 161, 247

Cancer*Care*, 192, 277

cancer cells, 5–6, 36; antigens produced by, 63; blood supply of, 36, 63; chemotherapy effects on, 36, 46–47, 48, 49; degree of differentiation of, 6; estrogen effects on, 142; growth/replication of, 36, 48–49; histologic types of, 6, 9, 208; immune system and, 64; residual, 36, 57; sanctuaries for, 108; seeding of, 33

Cancer Genetics Network, 16

Cancer Hope Network, 192

Cancer Support Community, 277

cannabinoids, 83

CA-125 serum level, 20, 25, 49, 56; before/during chemotherapy, 50, 56; to monitor treatment response, 52; in recurrent disease, 214, 234; screening of, 15–16, 17; surveillance after treatment completion, 213–14, 217–18, 232

capecitabine (Xeloda), 76, 91, 101, 247

carbohydrates, 55, 96, 111, 118, 172

carboplatin, 46, 50, 53, 59, 72

carboplatin/docetaxel doublet, 59, 243, 247

carboplatin/gemcitabine doublet, 59, 241–42, 244, 247

carboplatin/paclitaxel doublet, 241–43, 247

carboplatin/pegylated liposomal doxorubicin (PLD) doublet, 241–44, 247

carboplatin side effects, 242, 243–44; allergic reaction, 242; hand-foot syndrome, 243; infusion reactions, 103; lowered blood cell counts, 76, 85, 242, 244; nausea/vomiting, 85, 242; peripheral neuropathy, 97; in recurrent disease, 242–44

carcinoma, ovarian, 6, 30. *See also* epithelial ovarian cancer

carcinomatous ileus, 250

cardiopulmonary resuscitation/support, 263, 268

cardiovascular health and disease, 7, 27, 111, 140, 161, 167, 227–28; Avastin effects on, 245

care, survivorship, 138–54; for cognitive/memory changes, 149–51; complementary and alternative medicine, 146–47; for menopausal symptoms, 139–45; mind-body wellness, 151–52; plans for, 138, 219–20; for sleep disturbances, 147–49; surveillance, 216–19; theory of inner strength, 152–53

caregiver burden, 134–35

cells: growth/replication of, 36, 48–49; life span of, 5–6, 49

central access catheter, 50–51, 81

Cephulac (lactulose), 88, 89, 125, 134

cervical cancer, 14, 19, 228

"chemo-brain," 99–100, 149–51, 178–79, 180, 222–23

chemotherapy, 2, 35, 48–49, 138; baseline tests before, 50; cell susceptibility to, 36; central access catheter for, 50–51; changing drugs for, 52; complete clinical remission after, 49; consolidation, 56–57; day of administration of, 53; debulking surgery and effectiveness of, 36; definition of, 46; doctor visits before, 56; for epithelial ovarian cancer, 49–64; front-line, 49–56; immune function during, 113; intraperitoneal (IP), 37–38, 50, 51; intravenous/intraperitoneal (IV/IP), 50, 53–54; investigational drugs and clinical trials, 65–71; neo-adjuvant, with interval debulking, 38–39, 52, 54; for non-epithelial ovarian cancer, 65; nutrition and, 53, 55, 114–18; optimal, 47; preparing for next cycle of, 56; salvage, 56, 57–59; schedule for, 51–52; tests to predict effectiveness of, 235; tumor resistance to, 36, 39, 107. *See also specific drugs*

chemotherapy for recurrent disease, 57–59, 234–36, 241–48, 253; bevacizumab, 63, 244–45, 247; choosing based on side effects, 242–44; delay of, due to surgery, 237, 241; maintenance therapy, 244–45; olaparib, 245–46; platinum doublets, 241–44, 247; platinum-free interval and, 235–236, 237, 241; platinum-refractory cancer, 236, 238; platinum-resistant cancer, 233, 246–47; platinum-sensitive cancer, 233, 236–46, 247; regimens and cycles of, 241, 244

chemotherapy side effects, 49, 50, 54–55, 59, 74–105, 231; cognitive changes, 99–100, 149–51, 178–79, 180, 222–23; constipation, 72, 87–90, 115; diarrhea, 90–92; drug selection for recurrent disease based on, 242–44; fatigue, 54–55, 72, 94–97, 221; hair loss, 3, 55, 73, 75, 92–94; hand-foot syndrome, 100–102, 243; hearing loss, 55, 75; infusion reactions, 102–4; long-term and late effects, 221–23; low platelet count/bleeding, 73, 80–81, 85,

cyclo-oxygenase-2 (COX-2) inhibitors, 101, 102
cyclophosphamide (Cytoxan), 76, 82, 92, 247
cyclosporin, 161
Cylert (pemoline), 136
cytoreductive surgery, 34–38; neo-adjuvant chemotherapy and interval debulking, 38–39; secondary (repeat), 40–41, 58–59, 236–38
cytostatic agents, 46–47, 48
cytotoxic agents, 46, 48, 54, 58
Cytoxan (cyclophosphamide), 76, 82, 92, 247

dairy products, 91, 92, 114, 117, 118, 119, 120, 163
dancing, 146, 175, 253
debulking surgery, 34–38; interval, neo-adjuvant chemotherapy with, 38–39, 52, 54; secondary (repeat), 40–41, 58–59, 236–38
Decadron (dexamethasone), 83, 85
decision making, 3, 231; about chemo-therapy, 47, 58; about clinical trial participation, 68–69, 71; designating surrogates for, 264
decisions at end of life, 257–65, 270; alertness vs. pain relief, 262–63; com-munication for, 258–59; funeral/wake/celebration, 264–65, 270; intuba-tion/cardiopulmonary resuscitation, 262–64; legal documents for, 264; per-sonal perspectives on, 252–56; what to do with remaining time, 259–61; where and with whom to spend remaining time, 259, 262–65
definition of ovarian cancer, 5–6
dehiscence, 239
dehydration, 96, 178; ascites drain-age and, 251; chemotherapy and, 53, 82, 86, 115; cognitive effects of, 150; fatigue and, 95, 96, 178; IV fluids for, 82; prevention of, 86, 88; signs of, 86, 91–92; after surgery, 44. See also hydra-tion/fluid intake
Delestrogen (estradiol valerate), 143
dental care, 72, 77, 81
depression, 96, 100, 114, 136, 146, 150, 153, 193, 223–24, 231, 275; employment and, 225; exercise for, 146, 226; fa-tigue, chemo-brain and, 147, 150, 178, 188, 221; immune function and, 174;

insomnia and, 136, 222; integrative ap-proaches to, 176; medications for, 136; menopause and, 139; spiritual well-being and, 175; symptoms of, 136
dexamethasone (Decadron), 83, 85
dextroamphetamine (Dexedrine), 136
diabetes, 27, 39, 97, 112, 228, 243
diagnosis, 7, 23; differential, 24; of recur-rent disease, 233–34; symptoms and, 17–20, 24, 26; tests for, 24–27
diaphragm, tumor nodules on, 37
diarrhea: C. difficile, 240; chemotherapy-induced, 90–92, 96, 114; diet for, 45, 92, 116, 117; drug-induced, 83, 84, 129; medications for, 91, 92; patient educa-tion for, 91–92
diazepam (Valium), 83
diet. See nutrition/diet
dietary supplements, 29, 81, 87, 98, 118, 119, 120, 143, 145, 148, 151, 157, 159–62, 164, 172, 180; antioxidants, 119, 157, 164, 167–68; for bone health, 187; drug interactions with, 161, 180; for fatigue and chemo-brain, 179; FDA regula-tion of, 159–60; food components and natural products, 168–71; for hair and nail growth, 184, 185; for hot flashes, 177; for sleep, 176–77; vs. whole foods, 166–67. See also nutrition/diet
dietitians, 115–16, 117, 162
differentiation of cancer cells, 6
digitalis, 161
digoxin, 81
diphenhydramine (Benadryl), 54, 83
diphenoxylate and atropine (Lomotil), 92
disability benefits, 135, 192, 194, 204, 255
disease status, 68, 183, 216, 218, 233, 252
diverticulitis, 18, 24, 26, 218
dizziness, 79, 80, 91, 96, 97; drug-in-duced, 83, 127, 129
DNA (deoxyribonucleic acid), 49, 107, 176, 200–202, 209, 245
docetaxel (Taxotere), 76, 93, 97; with carboplatin for recurrent disease, 59, 243, 247
docusate sodium (Colace), 88
dolasetron (Anzemet), 83, 84
donation of body parts, 270
dong quai, 161
do not resuscitate order, 263
Doxil. See doxorubicin, pegylated lipo-somal

doxorubicin (Adriamycin), 72, 73, 76, 247
doxorubicin, pegylated liposomal (PLD; Doxil), 59, 67; with carboplatin for recurrent disease, 241–44, 247; for platinum-resistant recurrence, 247; shortage of, 243–44; side effects of, 73, 76, 91, 101, 185, 243
driving, 43–44, 54, 80, 97, 121, 173, 194
dronabinol (Marinol, THC), 83
droperidol (Inapsine), 83
drug resistance, 36, 39, 107
dry mouth, drug-induced, 83
Dulcolax (bisacodyl), 88, 89
durable power of attorney for health care, 264
dying and death, 1–2, 7; alertness vs. pain relief for, 262–63; brain death, 267–68; choosing where to die, 262; dealing with loss, 266–71; decisions at end of life, 257–65, 270; determination of death, 266, 267–68; with dignity, 253, 254, 256; disclosing to patient, 259–60; doctors' responses to, 270; fear of, 136, 255, 268–69; at home, 262, 263–64; personal perspectives on, 252–56; "silent killer," 18; support groups for, 256; during surgery, 13; withdrawal of cardiopulmonary support, 268
Dying Shame, 256
dysgerminoma, 65, 109
dyspareunia, 19, 141, 145, 222

early-stage ovarian cancer, 2, 25, 31, 227
eating difficulty, 18, 19, 20, 82, 86, 111, 114
echinacea, 161
echocardiogram, 27
economic issues, 135, 159, 192, 225; cost of pain medications, 123, 125; socioeconomic status and cancer risk, 10, 11. See also financial concerns; insurance, health
Effexor (venlafaxine), 129, 144, 177
electrocardiogram, 27, 267
electrolyte imbalances, 92, 96
Eloxatin (oxaliplatin), 76, 82, 97, 103
Emend: IV (fosaprepitant), 84; oral (aprepitant), 84
employment, 95, 97, 135, 192, 224–25, 255, 272; Family and Medical Leave Act, 192; protection against genetic discrimination, 204; returning to work, 183–84, 188, 192, 225
empowerment, 4, 35, 132, 154, 190, 195, 220

emtansine, 63
end of life: decisions at, 257–61, 270; hospice care for, 58, 249, 253, 262; palliative care and, 249–51; palliative surgery and, 41–42, 258; personal perspectives on, 252–56. See also decisions at end of life; dying and death
endometrial cancer, 7, 60, 227; diet and, 163–64, 165, 168; Lynch syndrome and, 209–10; tamoxifen-related, 228
endometrioid ovarian cancers, 6, 9, 60, 61
endometriosis, 9, 15
endoscopic retrograde cholangiopancreatography (ERCP), 26
endoscopy, gastrointestinal, 26
enemas, 28, 81, 88, 89–90, 125
energy: anemia and, 80; decreased (see fatigue); depression and, 136; diet and, 117–18; exercise and, 187; functional recovery and, 187–88; nausea/vomiting and, 82; supplements for, 169–71
energy medicine, 157
ephedra, 161
epidemiology, 7
epidermal growth factor receptor inhibitors, 64
epidural analgesia, 130
epinephrine, 174
epithelial inclusion cysts, 8–9
epithelial ovarian cancer, 6; antibody therapy for, 62–64; CA-125 level in, 15; chemotherapy for, 49–64; fertility and, 30; hormonal therapy for, 59–61; immunotherapy for, 64; origin of, 8–9; recurrence rate of, 107; symptoms of, 18; targeted biologic therapy for, 62; Type I and Type II tumors, 6, 7
erythropoiesis-stimulating agents (ESAs), 79, 80
esterified estrogens (Menest), 143
Estrace (micronized estradiol), 142
estradiol transdermal (Alora, Climara, Menostar, Minivelle, Vivelle Dot), 143
estradiol valerate (Delestrogen), 143
Estring (vaginal estrogen), 143
estrogen, 5, 10, 13; menopause and, 139–41
estrogen replacement therapy, 13, 140–43, 145, 197
estropipate (estrogen sulfate; Ogen, Ortho-Est), 142
ethinyl estradiol (Gynodiol), 143
etoposide (VP-16), 76, 93, 247
euphoria, drug-induced, 83

evening primrose, 161
exemestane (Aromasin), 61
Ex-Lax (senna), 72, 88, 89, 134

fallopian tube(s), 8, 9, 141; prophylactic
  removal of, 9, 13–14
Familial Ovarian Cancer Registry, 277
family and friends, 21–22, 116, 134–35,
  194–95
Family and Medical Leave Act, 192
family history: BRCA gene mutations
  and, 198–99, 207, 208–9; gathering information on, 204–7; Lynch syndrome
  and, 210; ovarian cancer and, 10–11,
  12, 17, 198–99, 201–7, 211; Peutz-Jeghers syndrome and, 211
family tree, 206–7
fatigue, cancer-related (CRF), 19, 94–95,
  178–79, 187–88, 221; anemia and, 78,
  96, 147, 178, 221; antiemetic-induced,
  84; chemotherapy-induced, 54–55, 72,
  94–97; exercise for, 95, 96, 179, 180, 187,
  221; integrative approaches to, 176,
  179; radiation-induced, 95; sleep and,
  147–48
fats, dietary, 55, 111, 114, 117, 118, 119–
  20, 156, 164, 172, 173
fear. See anxiety/fear
fecal impaction, 91
feeding tubes, 116–17
Femara (letrozole), 61
fentanyl, transdermal, 127
fertility-preserving surgery, 30–31
fever, 76, 77, 78, 91, 103
feverfew, 161
Fiberall (psyllium), 88
FiberCon (polycarbophil), 88
fiber in diet, 87, 88, 90, 92, 118, 119, 134,
  164, 250
"fight-or-flight" system, 173–74
financial concerns, 95, 135–36, 148, 182,
  192, 195, 224, 225–26, 274; bankruptcy,
  195, 225; inability to afford pain medications, 123, 125; resources for, 192,
  225–26; unemployment, 135, 182, 225.
  See also insurance, health
Financial Guidance for Cancer Survivors and
  Their Families: Off Treatment, 225
fish and fish oil, 117, 118, 119, 161–62,
  163, 164, 169, 173
fistulae, 41, 248
5-FU (fluorouracil), 91, 100, 101
5-HT$_3$ antagonists, 83, 84–85, 87
flaxseed, 120, 161, 173, 177–78

Fleet enema, Fleet Phospho-Soda (sodium phosphate), 88
fluids. See hydration/fluid intake
fluorouracil (5-FU), 91, 100, 101
fluoxetine, 177, 178
fosaprepitant (IV Emend), 84
friends. See family and friends
From Cancer Patient to Cancer Survivor: Lost
  in Transition, 215
"front-butt," 181
fruits. See vegetables and fruits
functional recovery, 187–88, 224–26
funeral/wake/celebration, 264–65, 270
furosemide, 81

gabapentin (Neurontin), 129, 144–45
garlic, 161
gemcitabine (Gemzar), 72, 76; with carboplatin for recurrent disease, 59, 241–
  42, 244, 247; for platinum-resistant
  recurrence, 247
gene mutations, 11, 201–12; BRCA, 9,
  11, 12, 198–99, 207–9, 210, 233, 245–46;
  inheritance of, 202–3; Lynch syndrome
  and, 209; Peutz-Jeghers syndrome and,
  210–11; research studies of, 211. See
  also hereditary ovarian cancer
genes, 200–201; oncogenes, 11; tumor
  suppressor, 11, 49, 202, 207
genetic counseling, 199, 203
Genetic Information Nondiscrimination
  Act (GINA), 204
genetic testing, 200–212; for BRCA gene
  mutations, 208–9; for Lynch syndrome, 210; for panel of genes, 211–12;
  personal perspective on, 198–99; for
  Peutz-Jeghers syndrome, 211; protection against discrimination based on,
  203–4
germ cell tumors, 6–7; chemotherapy for,
  65; radiation therapy for, 65, 108–9
ginger, 161, 179
gingko biloba, 161
ginseng, 161, 171, 179
glutamine, 73, 98
glutathione, 98, 223
goldenseal, 161
gonadotropin-releasing hormone agonists, 31
granisetron (Kytril), 83, 84
green tea, 161, 170
guided imagery, 148, 153, 157, 174, 175,
  176, 177, 179
gynecologic malignancy, 6

puncture for, 87, 160, 179; anticipatory, 82, 84; chemotherapy-induced (CINV), 3, 55, 73, 82–87; delayed, 82, 85–86; due to bowel obstruction, 87; due to infusion reaction, 103; integrative approaches to, 176, 179; medications for, 42, 53, 55, 73, 82–86, 87, 133; nutrition and, 114–15; patient education for, 86–87; PEG tube for, 42

Navelbine (vinorelbine), 76, 87, 97, 247

Neulasta, 73

Neupogen, 73

neurokinin-1 receptor antagonists, 84, 85

Neurontin (gabapentin), 129, 144–45

Neuropathy Association, The, 278

neutropenia, 75–77

no evidence of disease (NED), 49, 56, 57, 181, 183, 216, 232, 252–53, 274. *See also* remission

non-epithelial ovarian cancers, 6–7, 47; chemotherapy for, 65; in Peutz-Jeghers syndrome, 210

nonsteroidal anti-inflammatory drugs (NSAIDs), 128, 129

norepinephrine, 174

NRG Oncology, 15

numbness/tingling in fingers or toes, 75, 97, 98, 223, 242

nutrition/diet, 7, 110–21, 253; achieving and preserving adequacy of, 113–18; for anemia, 80; anti-inflammatory diet, 21, 157, 161, 172, 173; BRAT diet, 45, 92, 125; caloric intake, 29, 36, 111, 114, 115–18, 121, 163, 186, 250; cancer outcomes and, 156–58; for carcinomatous ileus, 250; after chemotherapy, 55, 117–18; before chemotherapy, 53; during chemotherapy, 114–17; considering approaches to, 162; for constipation, 44, 90, 124–25, 134; deficiencies in, 97, 111, 112, 114, 162; for diarrhea, 45, 92, 116, 117; fatigue and, 95, 96; food shopping and meal preparation, 116; Mediterranean diet, 157, 163–64, 165; for nausea, 86; nutritional plan, 115–16; recommendations for, 117, 118–20; snacks, 116, 173; "super foods," 168; support of, 29, 39, 41, 110, 113–14, 117, 186; surgery and, 29, 44–45, 112–13; after treatment completion, 226–27; whole foods vs. supplements, 166–67, 180 (*see also* dietary supplements); wound healing and, 112. *See also* specific food groups

nutritionists, 21, 115, 162

nuts and seeds, 88, 118, 120, 163, 164, 165, 169, 173

obesity/overweight, 7, 111, 112, 117, 172, 226–27, 239

occupational therapy, 99, 223

Ogen (estropipate), 142

oils in diet, 44, 120, 161–62, 163, 164, 165, 173

olaparib (Lynparza), 245–46

omega-3 fatty acids, 120, 161, 163, 164, 172–73, 178

omega-6 fatty acids, 172–73

omentum, removal of, 36–37

oncogenes, 11

Oncology Nursing Society, 278

Oncovin (vincristine), 97

ondansetron (Zofran), 73, 83, 84, 133

oophorectomy, 141, 205; prophylactic, 9, 12–13, 17

oral contraceptive pills (OCPs), 11, 12, 31, 161

Oregon Death with Dignity law, 253, 254, 256

origin of ovarian cancer, 8–9

Ortho-Est (estropipate), 142

orthosilicic acid (Biosil), 185

osteoporosis, 120, 140, 141, 144, 187

OVA1 blood test, 25

Ovarian Cancer Canada, 278

Ovarian Cancer National Alliance (OCNA), 192, 278; Survivors Teaching Students program, 189

Ovarian Cancer Network, 17

Ovarian Cancer Research Fund (OCRF), 278

Ovarian Cancer Research Program, 189

ovarian cysts, 16, 24, 31, 33

ovaries, 5; metaplastic cells in, 8; prophylactic removal of, 9, 12–13, 17; removal of, 141, 205

ovulation, 5, 8, 10, 11, 12, 31

oxaliplatin (Eloxatin), 76, 82, 97, 103

oxycodone, 127

paclitaxel (Taxol), 46, 52, 72; administration of, 53; with carboplatin for platinum-sensitive recurrence, 241–43, 247; failure to respond to, 52, 67; IV/IP therapy with cisplatin, 50, 53–54; for non-epithelial ovarian cancers, 65; for platinum-resistant recurrence, 247; for salvage therapy, 59

Library of Congress Cataloging-in-Publication Data
A guide to survivorship for women who have ovarian cancer / edited by Robert E. Bristow, MD, MBA, FACOG, FACS, Terri L. Cornelison, MD, PhD, FACOG, F.J. Montz, MD, KM, FACOG, FACS. — Second edition.

    pages   cm. — (A Johns Hopkins press health book)

    Includes bibliographical references and index.

    ISBN 978-1-4214-1753-0 (hardcover : alk. paper) — ISBN 978-1-4214-1754-7 (pbk. : alkaline paper) — ISBN 978-1-4214-1755-4 (electronic) — ISBN 1-4214-1753-7 (hardcover) — ISBN 1-4214-1754-5 (pbk. : alk. paper) — ISBN 1-4214-1755-3 (electronic) 1. Ovaries—Cancer—Popular works. I. Bristow, Robert E., editor. II. Cornelison, Terri Lynn, editor. III. Montz, Fredrick J., editor.

    RC280.O8M66 2015

    616.99'465—dc23   2014043209